THE **ALGAE OIL**
REVOLUTION

THE **ALGAE OIL** REVOLUTION

Fight Disease and Promote Brain Development and
Mental Health with the Vegan Elixir from the Sea

Michael Nehls, MD, PhD

Translated by Andy Jones Berasaluce

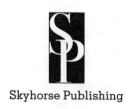

Skyhorse Publishing

Skyhorse Publishing books may be purchased in bulk at special discounts for sales promotion, corporate gifts, fund-raising, or educational purposes. Special editions can also be created to specifications. For details, contact the Special Sales Department, Skyhorse Publishing, 307 West 36th Street, 11th Floor, New York, NY 10018 or info@skyhorsepublishing.com.

Skyhorse® and Skyhorse Publishing® are registered trademarks of Skyhorse Publishing, Inc.®, a Delaware corporation.

Visit our website at www.skyhorsepublishing.com.
Please follow our publisher Tony Lyons on Instagram @tonylyonsisuncertain.

10 9 8 7 6 5 4 3 2 1

Library of Congress Control Number: 2024949280

Images on pages xiv, 4, 6, 10, 19, 21, 31, 32, 34, 39, 42, 43, 45, 48, 55, 58, 77, 105, 110, 127, 155, 159, 162, 174, 176, 178, 186: Shutterstock
Image on page 8: ID96097368 © Pglazar/Dreamstime.com
Image on page 184, left: NM Farm4, David Butaro, 2012 for Sapphire Energy
Image on page 184, right: Qualitas 2, Ryan Reid, 2016 for Qualitas Health
Images on page 185: Subitech GmbH
All other images and illustrations: courtesy of the author

Cover design by David Ter-Avanesyan
Cover image credit: Getty Images

Print ISBN: 978-1-5107-8306-5
Ebook ISBN: 978-1-5107-8307-2

Printed in the United States of America

For my parents

DISCLAIMER

All contents of this book have been researched and carefully checked to the best of our knowledge and belief, using sources that the author and publisher consider trustworthy. Nevertheless, as the author expressly notes, this book is not a substitute for individual medical advice. If you wish to seek medical advice, please consult a qualified physician. Neither the publisher nor author are liable for any adverse effects related, directly or indirectly, to the information contained in this book.

The information provided in this book is designed to provide accurate and authoritative information with respect to the subject matter covered. This book is not meant to be used, nor should it be used, to diagnose or treat any medical condition. For diagnosis or treatment of any medical problem, consult your own physician. While every attempt is made to provide accurate information, the author or publisher cannot be held accountable for any errors, omissions, or material which is no longer up to date.

CONTENTS

INTRODUCTION

At the head of all understanding—is realizing what is and what cannot be, and the consoling of what is not in our power to change.
—Solomon ben Yehuda (1021–1070)

Human dignity is inviolable. This human right also includes the right to healthy physical and mental development, and thus to a basic supply of everything needed for this development, such as clean drinking water or pollutant-free air. Ignoring basic needs results in mental and physical developmental disorders, as well as chronic diseases. These plunge people into deprivation: their dignity is being compromised.

The substances that we must obtain through food consumption include certain building blocks of proteins (essential amino acids), a whole range of trace elements, and all vitamins. F-Vitamins play a special role, as do vegetable omega-3 and omega-6 fatty acids found in high concentrations in flaxseed (linseed). However, unlike all other vitamins (A, B, C, etc.), F-Vitamins were discovered not while investigating a human disease of deficiency, but rather while performing experimental malnutrition on rats. Due to an artificially induced fat-free diet, the animals died within a few months. Flaxseed, on the other hand, or the oil obtained from this plant, saved the animals from certain death.

But flaxseed oil only helps us humans a little in counteracting the health consequences of a lack of omega-3 fatty acids. This is due to our development history: Unlike rats, our Paleolithic ancestors were not only gatherers but also fishermen. They did not live, as is generally believed, as hunters and gatherers roaming the savannahs for food. Rather, they settled near the coast and ate mainly fish and shellfish. This way of life provided them with sufficient high-quality aquatic omega-3 fatty acids—in contrast to terrestrial omega-3 fatty acids, which are, biologically, virtually ineffective for us—and the aquatic omega-3 fatty acids were ultimately essential for developing the human brain's extraordinary performance.

In prehistoric times, these aquatic food sources were inexhaustible, so humans didn't need to develop the ability themselves to produce omega-3 fatty acids. Unlike rats, we cannot efficiently produce them from plant precursors like those found in flax and other land flora. The human Vitamin F is different from the rat's: to develop optimally, our organism—especially our brain—needs oil not from terrestrial plants, but from aquatic sources.

During humankind's evolution from the Paleolithic fisherman and gatherer to the Neolithic cattle breeder and farmer around ten thousand years ago, there was a substantial reduction in aquatic omega-3 fatty acid intake from food. The deficiency this caused was accompanied by a serious reduction in size of the human brain. Over the last century, the increased industrialization of our food production has led to a further, no less significant change in the human diet, resulting in an even greater shortage of vital aquatic omega-3 fatty acids and an absolute excess of omega-6 fatty acids, which are found in many edible oils and animal products. The imbalance of these two fatty acids seriously threatens our health in general, but especially our children's intellectual development. The decline in rational thinking, as well as emotional and social intelligence, can hardly be compensated for through nutrition later in life. The extent of the problem is also evident in the global rise of many developmental disorders and diseases caused by aquatic omega-3 deficiency. These include ADHD and autism, cardiovascular diseases (cardio and cerebral infarction), most common forms of cancer, along with allergies and asthma. Last but not least, fatigue syndromes, anxiety, and depression as well as Alzheimer's and other dementias warrant mentioning here. All of these diseases have developed into pandemics over the past decades.

As you continue reading, you will probably reflect on your own life story. With every scientific fact that I encountered on this topic, I asked myself what I could have done differently and better in my life, in my childhood and also later, when feeding my own children. Much of what I know now was unknown to me at the time, and certainly not known to my parents or grandparents. Therefore, blame is misplaced; instead, a good degree of serenity is needed: Serenity to accept the things we can no longer change. On the other hand, we also need courage: The courage to change what needs to be changed. This includes correcting further undesirable developments that threaten our own future and that of our children. However, wise decisions about what to change and how to proceed can only be made if we are willing to learn from the past. If we don't do this, the catastrophic development towards a society that is psychologically increasingly ill and spiritually impoverished will continue to intensify. There are certainly many reasons for this development, but one key factor is widely misunderstood—and this is exactly the subject of the book you now hold in your hands: It is mainly the lack of omega-3 fatty acids that leads to a lack of foresight and empathy.

The overfishing of the world's oceans, the increasing contamination of steadily declining fish stocks with toxic heavy metals, pesticides, and plastic particles, as well as the effects of climate change are depleting the natural sources of vital, bioactive aquatic omega-3 fatty acids. Already today, adequate supplies for 7.5 billion people are no longer guaranteed. The sea can no longer supply it. It is overburdened, overfished, and increasingly contaminated—and that will not change in the foreseeable future. Therefore, we must urgently look for an equivalent alternative. In this book, I will introduce you to a revolutionary food product that will help tackle this global problem: Omega-3-rich oil obtained from microalgae.

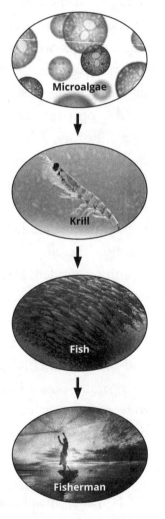

Microalgae

Krill

Fish

Fisherman

Microalgae are single-celled plants that are the only organisms capable of producing high-quality aquatic omega-3 fatty acids on their own. They just need light and carbon dioxide. As an essential part of the plankton, microalgae have been, since time immemorial, at the bottom of the aquatic food chain, which spans krill and fish, crabs and mussels, and at the top of which stand humans. As descendants of prehistoric fishers and gatherers, we owe the development of our extraordinary mental performance to the abundance of aquatic omega-3 fatty acids from microalgae. However, the advantage of an almost inexhaustible supply—at that time—of these brain-building materials also resulted in a biological dependence: We need aquatic omega-3 fatty acids in the same way we need oxygen to breathe, to stay mentally fit and physically healthy. The huge advantage of using microalgae directly to satisfy our needs for aquatic omega-3 fatty acids— rather than indirectly via fish and seafood—is that these algae can be produced in unlimited quantities, in a completely ecologically safe way. Because the oceans' capacity no longer suffices, this is the only cost-effective way to meet the entire world population's demand for high-quality, vital aquatic omega-3 fatty acids.

In addition, as a positive side effect, fish stocks could also recover.

We cannot turn the clock back to the Paleolithic period in order to live in a species-appropriate manner. Instead, we must venture forward into a (r)evolutionary future and diet that is eco-logically and economically sound and ethically harmless—and so sustainable that future generations can still inhabit our planet. Algae oil as a new staple is an important first step in this direc-tion. It is vegan, vital, and—I am convinced—totally without alternatives at present.

—Michael Nehls, July 2018

PART I

THE EVOLUTION OF THE HUMAN MIND

ENLIGHTENMENT FROM THE SEA

The longer you can look back, the farther you can look forward.
—Winston Churchill (1874–1965)

. . . And there was light.

However, for a long time no one was there to notice this—for a very long time, really.

After the force of gravity caused the sun to shine, it took about a billion years for the first microorganisms to colonize our planet's oceans. The Earth then orbited the Sun another two-and-a-half billion times until quite suddenly, about 540 million years ago, multicellular beings with eyes and a primitive nervous system emerged that could both see and process what they saw.

Within a relatively short period of about ten million years—more or less simultaneously, geologically speaking—almost all prototypes of today's animal kingdom developed. This "point" in geological history is called the Cambrian explosion. The term "cambrium" comes from *cambria*, the Latin name for Wales, where rock layers from that era were first examined in the 1830s.

Later, fossilized witnesses to this development were found in layers of earth around 500 million years old, in the Canadian Rockies' Burgess Shale.

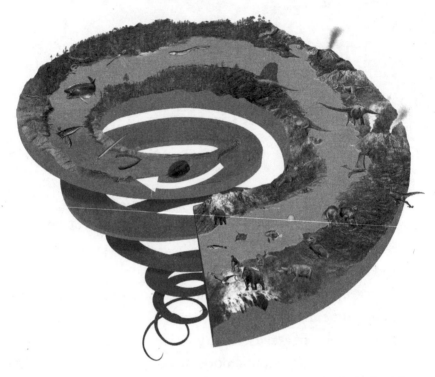

Almost all of today's animal phyla emerged during a relatively short time in the Cambrian period (arrow), about 500 million years ago.

The high speed at which new life developed so diversely at that time raises crucial questions: Why did it take so long for the light of creation to be seen? And above all, what made the emergence of life forms with increasingly complex nervous systems possible? These are questions that concern not only humanity's past, but also its future.

According to the usual explanation of the evolutionary process, all forms of life arise through random changes in genetic material, so-called mutations. Sometimes mutations give the genetically modified offspring an advantage: for example, the ability to see or slightly higher intelligence, resulting in better-adapted behavior.

Compared to living beings with unchanged genetic material, those with such beneficial mutations have an increased chance of passing on their "improved" (by virtue of being better adapted) genetic material to the next generation. This is called selection: mutations that improve the genetic material provide a selective advantage.

But does this evolutionary biological mechanism suffice to solve the mystery of the Cambrian explosion? After all, a dramatic development took place in just a few million years, which took several billion years to arrive. Something else must have enabled the evolution of sight and recognition.

Charles Darwin, the discoverer of the evolutionary principle, already suspected that the driving force in the emergence of completely new life forms cannot (only) be the interplay between mutation and selection: significant changes to the genetic material must also be preceded by serious environmental changes. Thus the question should be: What environmental changes allowed for the rapid emergence of a great diversity of species?

For a long time, due to the biosphere's chemical composition, our planet was too hostile for complex life. Because it lacked an ozone layer, the sun's UV radiation was able, unhindered, to sterilize the earth's surface. The oceans were also saturated with carbonic acid and toxic hydrogen sulfide and almost void of oxygen. As a result, life developed in the oceans in the form of rather primitive but quite robust microorganisms.

Science assumes that the Cambrian explosion was due to the increase in ocean oxygen levels, along with the simultaneous depletion of carbon dioxide, hydrogen sulfide, and many other toxic chemicals, which allowed aerobic organisms and increasingly complex life forms with high energy requirements to develop. The energy generated by an aerobic metabolism, i.e., one that uses oxygen, is almost twenty times higher than that generated by an anaerobic one, which doesn't use oxygen. Nervous systems are enormous energy guzzlers. Our brain, for example, based on its weight, needs over ten times more energy than the rest of our body.

Aquatic microorganisms, i.e., microorganisms living in water, were responsible for the serious change in these crucial environmental conditions. Their metabolism released oxygen as waste for many billion years. These microorganisms comprise both cyanobacteria, incorrectly called blue-green algae, and real, mostly single-celled microalgae, original forms of the plant world that emerged later (more on their origins in chapter 5). These primordial forms of life—cyanobacteria and microalgae—are still an essential part of plant plankton today and produce about half of the oxygen that we absorb through breathing.[1]

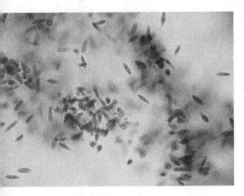

Plankton comprises all organisms living in the water whose swimming direction is predominantly determined by the current. The term derives from Ancient Greek and means "the wandering." Microalgae are an important representative of plant plankton.

With increased oxygen levels, evolution was able to produce a much more energy-efficient metabolism. This ultimately made even thinking of life possible. At the same time, however, this led to a dependency: our brain is the first organ to stop functioning without oxygen. You only have to hold your breath a moment to become aware of how dependent we are on plankton production even today.

Microalgae not only release oxygen, which is the energy supply for developing visual nervous systems, but also produce an indispensable building material: docosahexaenoic acid. This extraordinary fatty acid is also known as DHA. DHA belongs to the omega-3 fatty acids. We will look at their significance for our mental and physical health in more detail later. Briefly: without DHA from microalgae, the development of sight as we know it wouldn't have been possible—even today, this ability depends on DHA produced by microalgae. DHA finds its way to us mainly via fish and seafood, which is why it is referred to as an aquatic omega-3 fatty acid. It also is present in the flesh (meat) of terrestrial animals, although in much smaller quantities.

Sight occurs through communication between nerve cells. To perceive the visible world, light rays must be converted into nerve impulses. This is the responsibility of the visual sensory cells located in the eye's retina. As nerve cells, they are the part of the brain specialized in detecting light. Light sensors are embedded in their outer shell, known as the cell membrane, as shown in the following figure.

The light sensors are proteins that change their structure when light of a certain wavelength hits them. For this structural change to trigger an electrical nerve impulse so the incoming light can actually be perceived by the brain, DHA is required.[2] That is why DHA is found in high concentrations in the nerve cell membrane of the visual sensory cells. The light sensors are embedded in these DHA-rich sections of cell membrane.[3] For vision, the ability of DHA to take many very different spatial forms is of great importance.[4] As has been demonstrated experimentally, no other fatty acid, no matter how closely related, can replace DHA in this function.[5] Only DHA can be used to convert the light signal received from the light sensor into an electrical signal and transmit it as a neural impulse. Therefore, DHA is essential for vision.[6]

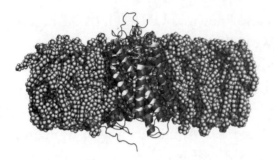

A section of the cell membrane of a visual sensory cell. Its outer shell consists of a double layer of fatty acids. Well over half of it is DHA. The light sensor is embedded in it.

Evolution also provides us with solid proof of DHA's exceptional position, as compared to other fatty acids: all vertebrate species examined so far, whether fish, amphibians, reptiles, or mammals, have the same—over 50 percent—exceptionally high concentration of DHA around their light sensors.[7] It is, therefore, clear that no other fatty acid has been able to prevail against DHA since the development of the common ancestor in the Cambrian explosion—despite Nature experimenting for over half a billion years. This finding has great clinical relevance: for example, infants need sufficient DHA from breast milk to develop good eyesight.[8] In addition, there are strong indications that aquatic omega-3 fatty acids protect against macular degeneration[9]— the leading cause of severe visual impairment and blindness in people over sixty years of age in the Western world.

FROM SEEING TO RECOGNIZING, THINKING, AND LEARNING

DHA is indispensable for converting light signals into electrical signals or nerve impulses for "communication" between our nerve cells and the outside world. It also has a similar function in perceiving what we see, i.e., in the communication between nerve cells. Here, too, a signal must be converted into an electrical impulse—again, impossible without DHA. This signal conversion takes place at the so-called synapses. Synapses form when the respective protrusions of two nerve cell membranes almost—and only almost—touch, as seen in the following figure.

The nerve cells exchange information across the gap aptly named the synaptic cleft. This works as follows: on one side, an electrical nerve impulse from the first nerve cell reaches its part of the synapse. This leads to the release of a neurotransmitter into the synaptic cleft. The neurotransmitter transmits the signal by traveling across the narrow cleft to the second nerve cell. There, the sensors (receptors) recognize the neurotransmitter and the neurotransmitter is converted back into an electrical nerve impulse, which is relayed to other areas of the brain or to muscle cells.

And here comes nature's trick that makes us feel and remember, think, plan, and act: the synapses decide whether there's a successful

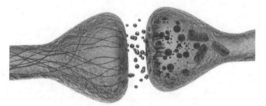

A synapse is the place where nerve cells communicate with each other by exchanging neurotransmitters.

signal transmission from one nerve impulse, via a neurotransmitter, to another nerve impulse. Previous signal transmissions determine the probability of future signals transmitting successfully or ending at the synapse. In this way, the synapses' behavior controls our behavior. Their ability to "calibrate," change, and adapt based on experience is called "synaptic plasticity." This is the basis for remembering or learning. More than a trillion synapses form the base of the complex human mind. The interplay of all these synapses, each of which is encoded within a tiny aspect of our accumulated life experience in a particular calibration, makes each of us unique. You could also say that we are our synapses: everything we see, what we feel, what we remember, our ideas, dreams, and desires—this is all the sum of our brain's synaptic processes.

Just as DHA is essential in converting a light signal into an electrical nerve impulse, this fatty acid is also crucial in synaptic signal transmission.[10] Accordingly, even the synapses' nerve cell membranes show an exceptionally high concentration of DHA of over 50 percent.[11] This is much higher than in the rest of the brain or other tissues.[12]

From a developmental perspective, DHA extracted from microalgae enabled the conversion of light signals into electrical nerve impulses. This particular fatty acid was also decisive for the evolution of other signaling systems, namely those of nervous systems, and, ultimately, of the human mind.[13]

The Versatile Brain Functions of DHA

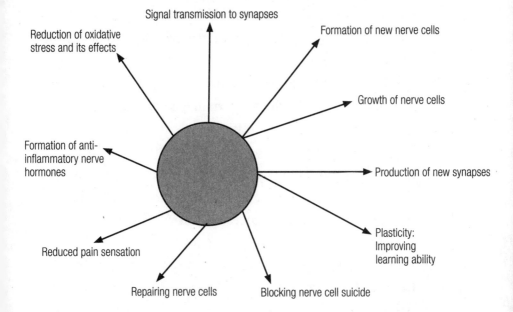

DHA isn't only building material for synapses, and it doesn't just enable communication between nerve cells. As the figure above shows, DHA is also a hormonal agent with functions as diverse as the complexity of its structure:

- DHA, as a hormone, stimulates the production of new nerve cells, a process called neurogenesis.[14] An adequate supply of DHA is therefore crucial for human brain growth during childhood.[15] Neurogenesis is also of exceptional importance for preserving memory and for mental well-being. In this context, it is referred to as adult neurogenesis.[16] It protects against depression[17] and—as I have shown—against Alzheimer's.[18] Activating adult neurogenesis is the most effective and, most likely, the only way to cure these two diseases.

- DHA stimulates nerve cell growth and new synapse formation.[19] Thus, this fatty acid hormone has enormous significance for the maturation of our emotional, social, and intellectual abilities.
- DHA prevents the death of nerve cells through various mechanisms when they are damaged by stress.[20] DHA makes nerve cells stress-resistant.
- DHA also supports the repair process.[21] With DHA administration following vertebral fractures or a stroke, there is much less permanent damage to the nervous system and the brain. Chances of recovery increased when DHA was administered.
- DHA reduces the pain sensation associated with chronic nerve cell damage or so-called neuropathic (nerve-derived) pain.[22]
- DHA inhibits oxidative stress, i.e., the harmful effect of excess oxygen radicals released due to inflammation or increased energy metabolism.[23]
- Last but not least, our organism uses DHA to form a number of other tissue hormones with a strong anti-inflammatory effect. Their task, after the causes of the damage have been eliminated, is to stop the inflammatory reaction and initiate repair of injured brain tissue.[24] With a chronic deficiency of DHA, both relative and absolute, there is a risk that the inflammation will become permanent, resulting in serious brain diseases.

DHA, therefore, plays an important role in the development and preservation of all mental functions, which leads to the following questions: If DHA has been essential for the mind's evolution since the Cambrian explosion more than half a billion years ago, why has no animal developed the ability to produce DHA on its own? Why are humans, in particular, presumably the most intellectually developed living being, dependent on a DHA supply from aquatic sources for life?

In fact, our metabolism is almost completely unable to efficiently produce DHA even from pre-prepared (plant-based) precursors. That is unusual. The example of arachidonic acid shows us an alternative. Arachidonic acid, abbreviated as AA, is an omega-6 fatty acid.

AA will be covered in more detail later because this fatty acid is as important and irreplaceable as DHA for mental development and maintaining our health.

However, there is no shortage of AA, unlike DHA, so we don't have to worry about sufficient supplies of this fatty acid. Even infants are able to produce AA from a plant-based omega-6 precursor up to a hundred times more efficiently than DHA from a corresponding omega-3 precursor, such as those found in flax and other plant sources.[25] The extremely low conversion rate of terrestrial omega-3 fatty acids in bioactive DHA is even further reduced in the presence of plant-based omega-6 precursors.

Fish and seafood, which were abundant throughout our evolution, are so rich in aquatic omega-3 fatty acids that our bodies never learned to produce them efficiently, even though we need them to survive.

Moreover, meat products, especially those from factory farms, contain virtually no DHA but a particularly high amount of prefabricated AA. If we are dependent on aquatic DHA, it's because we cannot produce it ourselves sufficiently. If we can metabolize AA from chemical precursors ourselves and there is more than

14

Terrestrial AA (arachidonic acid) is consumed almost daily by most people in the Western world in the form of meat and sausages.

enough available to us from terrestrial nutrition sources, then the crucial question arises: How did our Paleolithic ancestors, to whose way of life our metabolism is still adapted, feed themselves primarily—from aquatic or terrestrial sources? That is to say, more fish or more meat?

The classic picture we have of our prehistoric ancestors was described by science journalist Ann Gibbons, who specializes in human prehistory and early history, in 2002, for *Science* magazine. It shows "stocky hunters who bring wild animals home, divide their meat with stone tools and search the savannah for carcasses."[26] This picture of the so-called paleo-diet of Paleolithic hunters and gatherers, who fed themselves with plenty of meat as well as fruits and seeds, is also used to justify our modern diet with factory-farmed meat. Science tried to make this view plausible to us well into the last century.[27] But there is something wrong with this picture. To identify the problem, it helps to look at a fundamental evolutionary selection criterion: energy efficiency.

All living beings need sufficient energy. Those unable to get enough energy from food in the long-term risk losing their lives. Since there is always the danger of a food shortage, saving is a must. Accordingly, our metabolism naturally works as energy-efficiently as possible. This means that we do not ourselves generate all the products that we can easily acquire externally—that would be a waste of energy.

If an organism relies on food for its entire energy supply, it saves twice as much: on the one hand, it saves on producing these natural substances, and on the other, because it does not have to develop a complex biochemical production process solely to have energy available for life in case of an emergency. However, the advantage to saving energy in this way also has a disadvantage: lifelong dependence on external supply. Conversely, this means that whenever evolution failed to create the genetic prerequisites for the inherent ability to produce a vital food component when needed—such as vitamins— there couldn't have been, at least, a chronic shortage of any of these products. Otherwise, logically, the species could not have survived.

Based on these considerations, we can deduce something crucial about our ancestors' lifestyle and diet from the relative efficiency with which we can or cannot produce the two vital fatty acids, AA and DHA, from their precursors:

- Since we are extremely inefficient when it comes to DHA, this vital omega-3 fatty acid must always have been part of the Paleolithic basic diet.
- On the other hand, AA must have been in short supply, which is why its production from the corresponding (vegetable) omega-6 precursors is not only much higher but even favored.

Had humans actually been hunters-gatherers in the last phase of their development, which still characterizes us today, they would always have been abundantly supplied with terrestrial AA, but only inadequately with aquatic omega-3 fatty acids. This allows for only one conclusion: Our picture of the Paleolithic period is wrong! In this sense, Gibbons also arrives at a more accurate picture in the *Science* article cited above, namely "One of fishermen—and fisherwomen—who waded through calm lakes and carefully combed the shore for fish, eggs of seabirds, mussels, and other marine food."

ON FISHERMEN AND GATHERERS

Nutritionists at Imperial College in London have confirmed this thesis. According to their extensive research, the idea that "human evolution took its advantage from the marine [aquatic] food chain is irrefutably substantiated by fossil evidence."[28]

Crucial for the development of today's Homo sapiens sapiens—double sapiens, as we consider ourselves not just wise but "very wise"—was the discovery of high-quality, easy-to-digest, DHA-rich aquatic foods from inland freshwater, and above all, from coastal saltwater: fish, mussels, crabs, all of which are DHA concentrates.

Only through this aquatic type of nutrition did the human skull's volume grow to an all-time record size, from around two hundred thousand years ago to the beginning of the Early Stone Age around twelve thousand years ago.[29] Particularly crucial for this were the first fifty thousand years of this period. And there was a silver lining to our misfortune: misfortune because around 194,000 years ago, an ice age caused the central regions of Africa to become deserted. This period of drought lasted well over seventy thousand years and brought humanity slowly but mercilessly to the brink of extinction. Few survived. Genetic studies show that the development of today's human being was through a sort of bottleneck. According to genetic analysis, all representatives of different ethnicities come from only a few common ancestors—those who survived this long-lasting catastrophe.[30]

We were lucky, however, because the few hundred people able to save themselves by settling in coastal regions of southern Africa found a Garden of Eden. The Tree of Knowledge actually grew there, in the form of shell beds as far as the eye could see.[31]

Perhaps the omniscient God, contrary to what the Bible suggests, wanted us to eat of this "tree." At least the DHA-rich, and thus spirit-giving, seafood created the best conditions for a final growth spurt for a large, inquisitive brain—and for beginning the social conquest of the earth.

> Mussels feed on microalgae, which they filter from the sea. This makes them culinary DHA powerhouses.

In addition, the South African Cape is a unique floral kingdom due to its extensive and independent plant wealth. There, even our earliest relatives found countless plants with carbohydrate-containing roots, such as various species of the *fynbos* vegetation (Afrikaans for "bushes with fine leaves," derived from the Dutch *fijnbosch*), which also provided them with the plant precursor of AA.

Accordingly, Curtis Marean, professor of human evolution at Arizona State University in Tempe, and one of the discoverers of this Paleolithic Garden of Eden in which humanity survived and matured, writes: "Anyone who knows how to use a digging stick practically can't starve to death there."[32]

Over many thousands of generations, the genetic makeup of the people who survived in this area adapted to this spirit-enhancing diet of seafood and root vegetables. Even today, the diet is perfectly compatible with our basic genetic equipment. That's why it gives us the highest life expectancy, as an extensive study found.[33] The study showed that pescatarians, who consume fish and seafood in addition to vegetables, live much healthier and longer than people who instead regularly eat meat. Pescatarians also have an advantage over so-called lacto-vegetarians, who consume animal dairy products, and over vegans, who completely avoid fish and seafood.

This would seem to solve the mystery of the origin of man's extraordinary intellectual performance. Stephen Cunnane, physiologist at the University of Sherbrooke in Quebec, Canada, shares this view: "Once we [our ancestors] became able to exploit the coastal African food chain—far richer and more reliable than domestic sources of fish—brain development and cultural evolution exploded."[34]

Indeed, much of the evidence found in the caves on Africa's southeastern cape points to a much earlier evolution of the human mind than long assumed. For example, more than 164,000 years ago, people developed complex technologies such as the targeted heat treatment of stone materials to produce razor-sharp blades.[35] This required experience and planned action, along with complex language to pass on the acquired knowledge and skills to the next generations.

Large mounds of discarded shells, fish bones, and even technological artifacts have been found In South African caves —evidence of the existence of human communities, their settled lifestyle, and intellectual creativity dating back almost two hundred thousand years.

The inexhaustibility of local food sources led to sedentary behavior. A few hours a day were enough to get the daily requirement of seafood and nutritious root vegetables. This yielded more free time that could be used creatively. The abundance of food also allowed for an increase in the local population. This trend can be observed among all wild peoples, whether among the

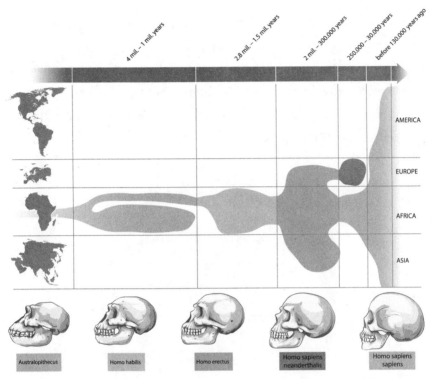

The cradle of humanity was in Africa. From there, our early ancestors, such as Homo erectus and Homo sapiens neanderthalis, moved out farther and farther. But it was only the "very wise" man, the homo sapiens sapiens, who succeeded in achieving the necessary intellectual breakthrough to enable him to subjugate the entire planet.

natives of Australia or those of North or South America: whenever a community fed mainly on aquatic sources instead of terrestrial ones, i.e., lived as fishers-gatherers instead of as hunters-gatherers, it grew.[36]

The larger the social groups that live closely together, the more frequently arise internal conflicts that need resolving, which requires emotional and social intelligence. At the same time, there's a sense of ownership because food sources must remain secure for one's own family. (For comparatively small communities still living today in nomadic ways, ownership is largely foreign.) However, the settled fisher and gatherer had to learn to exist within his own social structures and defend the common territory against the intrusion of foreign groups. This circumstance encouraged the evolution of cooperative behavior—a prerequisite for man's "social conquest" of the earth.[37]

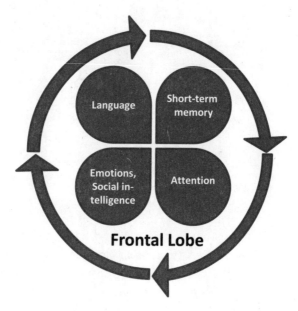

The interaction of executive functions of the human brain.

It is therefore not surprising that the frontal lobe, especially, increased in size compared to other brain regions. This part of the brain is the seat of our executive functions: where we plan, decide, and ultimately act.[38] The frontal lobe is also the center of our emotional and social intelligence, language, short-term or working memory, and attention, all of which are critical to cooperative behavior. It is not entirely by chance that the frontal lobe also contains the highest concentration of DHA in the entire brain.[39]

The frontal lobe also shows the greatest differences from the Neanderthal. The Neanderthal's frontal lobe was much less developed than the hindbrain, which housed his visual center.[40] It is believed that his brain was optimized for hunting, as his comparatively large eyes also indicate. His emotional and social skills, as well as his ability to speak, are likely to have been far less well-developed.

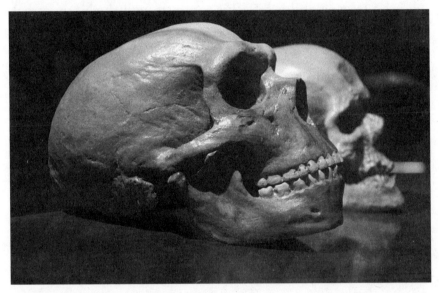

The Neanderthal's brain (skull in foreground) was optimized for hunting. His large eyes were connected to a large visual center (in the back of the skull). The brain of the modern human of the time (skull in background), on the other hand, had a large frontal lobe (forehead), optimized for all executive functions.

Meanwhile, increasing scientific evidence confirms an earlier assumption that our species, originating from Africa, conquered the earth primarily along its waterways.[41] This was the only way a growing population could obtain an adequate aquatic diet. The primary routes of dissemination were along the Nile, the waters of the Great Rift Valley, which stretches around four thousand miles from what is now Mozambique in the south to Syria in the north, or directly across the sea. According to the latest findings, our direct ancestors were already—130,000 years ago—capable of building boats and navigating the open sea.[42] Even back then, people were anything but primitive.

Until about twelve thousand years ago, the European descendants of South African fishers and gatherers primarily fed themselves on mussels and fish.[43] This contrasts with the Neanderthal, who, as a prototypical hunter, mainly fed on the meat of their prey[44]. The hunter was mentally inferior to the fisher and ultimately did not survive the competition.

The most recent bones and, thus, the last remains of Neanderthal life found, date back about thirty thousand years. This should give us pause, because after all, the majority of humanity today eats like the Neanderthals once did, i.e., the meat and plant products the land and soil provide. We have become domesticated hunter-gatherers without hunting or gathering ourselves. We leave these to the agricultural industry.

* * *

Modern humans are characterized by the development of a social-thinking, social-planning, and sociolinguistic brain: that of the Paleolithic fisher-gatherer. All the decisive factors for this evolution converged in South Africa's "Garden of Eden": the need for more complex social behavior, time for creative (symbolic) thinking and technological developments, as well as an almost inexhaustible source of aquatic food that provided enough essential brain-building materials.

But this shift towards greater social intelligence is not a one-way street. If you take away just one of these brain- and mind-shaping factors, the course reverses. A corresponding study published in 1997 in the renowned British science magazine *Nature* should make us all take notice: the human brain shrinks. Since switching from fishing and gathering to breeding livestock and cultivating fields, our mental development has been going backwards— at least insofar as brain size is a measure of mental potential.[45] According to this, since the transition from the Paleolithic fishing economy to the Neolithic agricultural economy, our brains have shrunk by an average of eleven percent.

Yuval Noah Harari, a history professor at the Hebrew University in Jerusalem, described this transition from fishing and gathering to a supposedly easier way of life as a farmer and livestock breeder as "the greatest fraud in human history,"[46] because it didn't really get any easier—rather, the opposite. Since then, our diet has been primarily terrestrial and less and less aquatic—and that didn't end well for the Neanderthals.

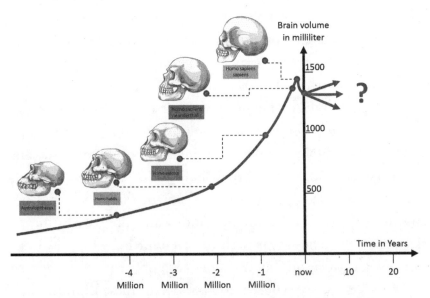

Where should humanity's spiritual journey go? Towards more or less potential?[47]

There are various explanations for the negative trend in mental development. Cell and developmental biologist Gerald Crabtree at Stanford University in California blames this on lower economic selection pressure, which increasingly enabled even less intelligent people to survive.[48] To survive, you have to live in a complex society based on the division of labor, its development determined by agriculture, making it possible to be far less mentally fit. As a result, according to Crabtree, there has since been a buildup of genetically harmful changes that have caused humans to lose some of their genetic potential in terms of brain size and intelligence.

Although Crabtree's arguments cannot be completely dismissed, I am convinced there are much more powerful forces that determine our mental fitness. The potential for brain growth is genetically determined.[49] However, how much of this potential can be used depends crucially on lifestyle, especially diet.[50] As you know, DHA stimulates new brain cell formation from infancy to old age. In doing so, it activates genes that make us mentally fitter and, in turn, switches off other genes whose function would have the opposite effect long-term.[51]

Consequently, a chronic shortage of aquatic omega-3 fatty acids, such as DHA, is enough to limit brain growth to only a small part of its potential and to limit its retention over the course of life. In fact, brain shrinkage continues to occur—and the cause is not genetic. Extensive studies have found that the lower the absolute and relative proportion of aquatic fatty acids in a person's diet, the smaller the brain.[52] At the same time, with omega-3 deficiency, the tendency is to shrink even further with age. This is not just a correlation, but a major cause of mental developmental disorders. As we will see in more detail, these disorders have been proven to simultaneously cause an increased risk of ADHD, autism, depression, and the most common forms of dementia. The pandemic increase of these diseases indirectly provides further evidence that our genetic makeup is still adapted to a lifestyle and diet rich in fish and seafood.[53]

In retrospect, it is likely that the Paleolithic fisher-gatherer was actually a double sapiens. Even today, we could make better use of our genetically available intellectual potential if we were to again eat a more species-appropriate diet. We therefore need not assume—unlike Crabtree—that we have lost this potential. I like this explanation because it gives us legitimate hope that we can counteract this trend of intellectual impoverishment through a few measures. The question that every person individually and society, as a whole, must ask is: Do we want to continue to eat more like Neanderthals, lots of meat and, therefore, a diet rich in AA and low in DHA, or, rather a diet rich in DHA and balanced in AA, like our intelligent ancestors?

However, a steadily increasing global shortage of this DHA brain elixir is still causing average mental fitness to become increasingly impaired. The danger of an intellectual, social, and emotional regression of the human spirit is all the more serious when one considers the enormous challenges humanity faces: pandemics of preventable diseases, globalization and digitalization, development of superhuman (post-human) artificial intelligence, environmental destruction as well as species extinction. Our survival in humane conditions is at stake, if not our very existence as a species.

Today's diet is characterized by meat products that are low in DHA and high in AA. This diet is based on industrial farming and the outdated and unfortunately very unhealthy notion that our Paleolithic ancestors were primarily hunters.

Given these dangers, a better understanding of our past can guide our future. This much we know for sure: The human spirit, like life itself, comes from the sea. Humans' social intelligence has allowed them to dominate the planet. But will this creative spirit be intelligent enough to preserve the basis of its existence?

With an eye towards our own health and tackling pressing future questions, we must strive to provide ourselves with adequate supplies of essential brain-building materials. To do this, we must first clear up historical errors, outdated doctrines and, not least, the market interests that harm consumers. It is, therefore, important to understand the world of vital fatty acids.

PART II

AN EXCURSION INTO THE WORLD OF FATTY ACIDS

IGNORANCE MAKES
YOU SICK

Let food be thy medicine, and let medicine be thy food.
—Hippocrates of Kos (460–370 BC)

For the sake of our own health alone, we should know and understand which fatty acids are healthy and which are not, why some are vital, and what role they play in our mental and physical well-being. We should also understand why some fatty acids must be consumed through food, while others are better avoided. However, this is hardly possible without a rough knowledge of their structure, which I'll try to represent simply here.

Knowledge of fatty acid structure is also a prerequisite for the ability to distinguish correct information from the nonsensical and deliberately incorrect—and that is vital. Only with proper knowledge can you see how the food industry, which is dominated by economic interests, is trying to manipulate its consumers with false messages. There is a lot of misinformation, and that, too, is calculated. When there is completely contradictory information on a certain topic everywhere, many people give up when just trying to work towards a healthy diet.

How are you supposed to distinguish sense from nonsense, or market interests from scientific facts? Especially since science isn't always credible, even when it purports to give pure facts.

According to expert Christian Kreiß, the food industry uses third-party funding to influence which questions are asked in university research and which answers are ultimately made public. I conclude that this influences statements of supposedly independent experts—and, in turn, steers public opinion.[1] This influence is understandable from corporations' perspective. Ultimately, they only win the market economic battle for survival through sales and profit optimization. The primary goal in producing many foods is not, a priori, to improve or maintain consumer health, but to achieve financial profit. For the same reason, politicians repeatedly pass laws that are primarily industry-friendly, even if they harm us consumers. The power of the economic giants and their lobbyists should not be underestimated.

A deeper look into the world of fatty acids will also help you understand the paradox of why a deficiency in essential fatty acids has been proven to lead to myriad very serious diseases, yet clinical trials often fail to provide the ultimate proof of their benefit for prevention or therapy. However, to understand this, we need some chemistry. But this should not deter the non-chemists among you. Chemistry is nothing more than a large construction toy kit with a little over a hundred different kinds of "LEGO bricks." To build and understand fatty acids, we only need three. Of course, the chemical LEGO bricks aren't square structures, but spherical: the white spheres are hydrogen atoms, the gray ones are oxygen atoms, and the black ones are carbon atoms. Besides color, the spheres differ in the number of plug-in options: hydrogen has one, oxygen two, and carbon even has four. Depending on how you put these spherical LEGO bricks together, you get compounds with completely different properties. But before we turn to the fatty acids, I'll first show you how to play "chemical LEGOS" with these three spheres using a few simple examples.

Water is created when two white spheres (hydrogen), are combined with a gray sphere (oxygen). Water was called hydro in ancient Greek, which is why chemical compounds that contain water are also called hydrates. For example, if you place a black sphere, i.e., carbon, between the gray sphere and one of the two white spheres that form water, or hydra, you get a so-called carbohydrate: a simple compound made of carbon and water.

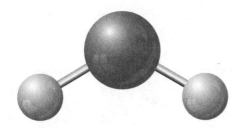

Water is a simple compound consisting of two hydrogen molecules and one oxygen molecule.

Water

Since carbon has four plug-in points, two of them remain unoccupied. Such unused plug points are typical of so-called radicals. If the other carbon slots remained unoccupied, we'd be dealing with a carbon radical. If it were oxygen instead of carbon, one would speak of oxygen radicals. Such oxygen radicals are released during inflammation and energy metabolism and are, therefore, very aggressive because they are looking for a partner with which they can connect. If it's the wrong one, tissue damage can occur.

With these simple carbon-in-water compounds, Nature solves the problem by stringing several of them together across the still-free connectors, like beads on a chain. Depending on how they are connected, they end up as something approximating a large ring. A typical representative is dextrose, also known as glucose.

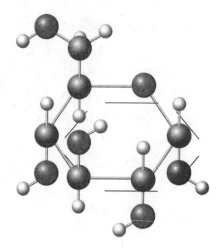

Glucose is a carbohydrate consisting of a chain of six carbon-in-water compounds that form a ring.

Glucose

Another example of such a somewhat more complex carbohydrate chain is fructose.

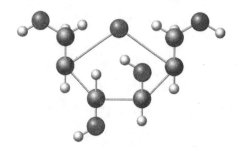

Fructose consists of almost the same number of building blocks as glucose; they are just arranged a little differently.

Fructose

As a look at these two "LEGO constructions" shows, glucose and fructose look almost the same, but not quite. They behave very differently chemically and, moreover, biologically. This is a typical effect that we will also see with fatty acids: small differences in chemical composition often have serious biological effects, and, by extension, health effects.

Fructose tastes much sweeter than glucose. Also, fructose is metabolized almost exclusively in the liver, which is associated with the risk of fatty liver and can also cause gout. In contrast, glucose is primarily converted, in fat cells, into so-called saturated fatty acids. In this form, the (chemical) energy stored in the sugar is available long-term, if needed. Saturated fatty acids are therefore important for maintaining our health.

SATURATED FATTY ACIDS— SIMPLE AND HEALTHY

There are many different fatty acids. They form a large family whose members are characterized by commonalities. These can be clearly seen in the figure below, using stearic acid as an example:

- Fatty acids consist of a chain of carbons.
- Each chain has two ends. These are referred to as alpha and omega, the first and last letters of the Greek alphabet.
- The carbon at the alpha end is linked to two oxygens. There is also a hydrogen molecule attached to one of the two oxygens. This or its core is readily released into water, when it is nearby. This process acidifies the water. The alpha end, thus, turns the fatty acid into an acid.
- The omega-end carbon has three hydrogens. This end is chemically neutral and, correspondingly, fat-soluble.

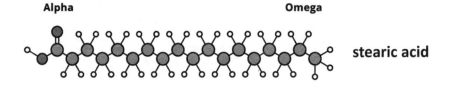

Alpha   **Omega**

stearic acid

Stearic acid is an example of a saturated fatty acid. With eighteen carbons in its chain, it is one of the most common fatty acids found in land-dwellers' stored fat.

As you can also see in the figure, stearic acid has two hydrogens on all carbons between the alpha and omega ends. Thus, this fatty acid is considered saturated: no hydrogen is missing.

This makes saturated fatty acids such as stearic acid chemically very stable, and well-suited for long-term energy storage and retention. That's why nature has designed it so we can produce unlimited quantities of saturated fatty acids from carbohydrates to store them in our fat tissue.

Saturated fatty acids have been falsely reputed to be unhealthy because most foods containing large amounts of saturated fatty acids, such as meat or dairy products, are unhealthy and daily consumption shortens life.[2] However, a fatty acid is never the only factor; other fatty acids and other food components can make these products harmful in one way or another. The assumption that saturated fatty acids cause diseases such as arteriosclerosis, as well as heart or cerebral infarctions has now clearly been refuted. It was based partly on incorrect data and partly on incorrect interpretations.[3]

Why should saturated fatty acids be unhealthy when nature's design for millions of years has been for us to produce them ourselves in large quantities, and store them for emergencies? After all, our metabolism is optimized for staying healthy and surviving, not for ailing and premature death. Only when the fatty tissue in the abdominal area, where saturated fatty acids are predominately stored, gets out of hand through so-called carbohydrate fattening, does it have a detrimental effect on health. However, this is not due to the stored fatty acids themselves but because our fatty tissue is hormonally active. If this "endocrine gland" grows to an unnatural size, like a kind of abdominal goiter, excess weight occurs—not just affecting the figure—due to producing and releasing its fatty tissue hormones. This mismanagement causes chronic inflammation, high blood pressure, diabetes, and a whole armada of other health problems.[4]

The erroneous idea that saturated fatty acids are inherently unhealthy is also disproved by recognizing that fasting is healthy, since it is precisely during this process that the fatty tissue releases large quantities of these supposedly unhealthy fatty acids. These, in kind, reach the liver via the blood and there are converted into ketone bodies. Ketone bodies are small fatty acid fragments which can easily reach the brain, where they supply it with valuable energy—even more effective than sugar.[5]

But this is not the only reason why fasting is so healthy. We now know that ketone bodies are more than brain food, they are hormone-like signaling substances. These stimulate processes that rejuvenate our brain cells[6] and stimulate the growth of our brain's memory center.[7] In 2016, the Nobel Prize in Medicine was awarded in recognition of the rejuvenating and health-promoting effects of fasting. Saturated fatty acids are not only completely harmless from a medical perspective, but also extremely healthy due to their many important biological functions.

This is especially true for coconut oil because it consists mainly of saturated fatty acids. These are mainly medium length (ten to fourteen carbons) and are—in contrast to longer fatty acids from other plant and animal sources—transported to the liver directly after digestion. In this way, they bypass storage in fat cells. Instead, they are converted by the liver cells into healthy ketone bodies. Another important property of saturated fatty acids is visible to the naked eye in native coconut oil: its high melting point

Native coconut oil is spreadable at room temperature due to its naturally high content of saturated medium-chain fatty acids.

turns the oil into solid fat when it cools to room temperature (75.2° Fahrenheit/24° Celsius and colder).

The reason can be seen in the earlier example of stearic acid. As in that situation, the two hydrogens, each attached to a carbon within the carbon chain, mutually avoid their "neighbors": there are always two hydrogens arranged alternately at the top and again at the bottom. As a result, the saturated fatty acid takes on a zigzag shape and becomes elongated. This allows saturated fatty acids to stick well together along their entire length, leading to the solidification of the oil.

UNSATURATED FATTY ACIDS—COMPLEX AND HEALTHY

If not all the carbons within the carbon chain have two hydrogens attached, then the entire fatty acid is considered unsaturated. It could potentially absorb more hydrogen molecules until it finally becomes saturated.

Because the "LEGO carbon spheres" have four insertion points and all are used for stability, unsaturated carbons always appear as adjacent pairs. The remaining free plug-in point is used for a second connection between the two neighboring carbons. Such unsaturated pairs are linked by two dashes instead of a single line in schematic representations, like the figure below. The double line represents a so-called double bond and is an indication of an unsaturated fatty acid.

The first unsaturated carbon pair counted from the omega end is characteristic of a certain class of unsaturated fatty acids. Oleic acid is, therefore, an omega-9 fatty acid. As can also be seen in the figure, the individual hydrogens of the unsaturated carbon pair are located on the same side of the fatty acid, or double line. This is why it is a so-called cis fatty acid. If they were opposite each other, it would be a trans fatty acid (more on that later).

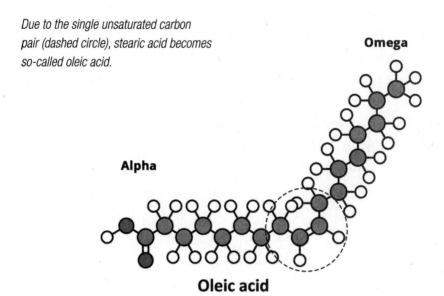

Due to the single unsaturated carbon pair (dashed circle), stearic acid becomes so-called oleic acid.

Omega

Alpha

Oleic acid

This distinction between cis fatty acid and trans fatty acid is enormously important. Only when the two hydrogens are arranged in the cis position does the fatty acid get "kinked" (with trans fatty acids, it remains stretched, as we'll also see later). Because of the kink, cis fatty acids can no longer attach themselves to each other lengthwise. This means that much less heat is required to melt oils that consist primarily of "kinked" fatty acids. In contrast to oils made primarily from saturated fatty acids (or trans fatty acids), these are usually still liquid even at cooler temperatures.

All natural human foods contain cis fatty acids, which is why our organism struggles with trans fatty acids when they enter our diet. (We will discuss this in more detail shortly.)

Cis fatty acids are preferably incorporated into cell membranes, where they ensure that membranes are not rigid, but rather highly

Olive oil is primarily composed of monounsaturated cis oleic acid. As a result, olive oil remains liquid even in the refrigerator.

flexible. This flexibility is also called fluidity. It gives all components in biological membranes the ability to move more freely within them and thus come into better contact with one another.

Our organism can produce omega-9 fatty acids like oleic acid, simply by completely removing the corresponding two hydrocarbons from stearic acid. For this "desaturation," so-called desaturases are responsible.

The essential F-vitamins for rats were discovered in flaxseed oil. It contains approximately 15 percent oleic acid and linoleic acid (LA), as well as—extraordinary for plant oils—70 percent alpha-linolenic acid (ALA).

Desaturases are biochemical catalysts whose structure and function are determined in our genetic makeup. Since we have the blueprint for an omega-9 desaturase in our genome, omega-9 fatty acids are not an essential dietary component. We are not dependent on their supply, unlike polyunsaturated omega-3 and omega-6 fatty acids. Why? We lack a blueprint for omega-3 or omega-6 desaturase.

F-VITAMINS—
A HISTORICAL ERROR

Until the end of the 1920s, it was believed that fatty acids and carbohydrates (sugar and starch) were simply different energy sources—and thus interchangeable. A calorie from fatty acids was considered equivalent to a calorie from carbohydrates. It was thought that only the energy content mattered. But when the researcher couple Georg and Mildred Burr fed their laboratory rats a completely fat-free diet, they became ill and died within a few months—despite a sufficient caloric supply of carbohydrates.[8]

However, administering flaxseed oil saved the animals from certain death. Over the following decades, two life-saving fatty acids for rats were gradually isolated. Flax plants, which belong to the genus *linum*, also gave their name to the vitamins discovered: linoleic acid and alpha-linolenic acid.[9] After the previous discovery of vitamins A, B, C, D and E, these were called Vitamin F, also, appropriately, an abbreviation for fatty acid.

Alpha-linolenic acid (ALA) is an omega-3 fatty acid because the first unsaturated carbon pair is in the third position at the omega end, as shown in the figure below. Two more are in sixth and ninth positions. ALA is therefore a polyunsaturated fatty acid or, more precisely, a triple unsaturated (triunsaturated) fatty acid.

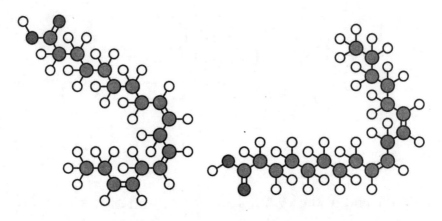

alpha-linolenic acid (omega-3)   **linoleic acid (omega-6)**

Left: Alpha-linolenic acid (ALA) is a triunsaturated omega-3 fatty acid. They are found in very high concentrations in flaxseed oil. Right: Linoleic acid (LA) is a diunsaturated omega-6 fatty acid. It is also contained in flaxseed oil. They are found in very high concentrations in most oils that dominate the modern Western diet.

Linoleic acid is abbreviated as LA. Starting at the omega end, it has the first unsaturated carbon pair in the sixth position, making it an omega-6 fatty acid. A second unsaturated carbon pair is in the tenth position. LA is, therefore, a diunsaturated fatty acid.

No animal can produce omega-3 and omega-6 fatty acids on its own. Even humans simply lack the desaturases suitable for removing hydrogen that is closer than the seventh position to the omega end. However, it was never necessary for the animal kingdom to develop these special tools, because plants produce ALA and LA to store energy, especially to supply the next generation, which is why seeds and nuts are enriched with these fatty acids.

Most seeds and their corresponding oils have a high to very high proportion of LA. Examples include sunflower, corn germ, soybean, or safflower oil. However, these are almost free of ALA.

Few plants produce relatively high amounts of ALA and store it in their seeds. Examples are flax, chia, walnut, or rapeseed. Otherwise, ALA can be found in leafy vegetables (cabbages) and salads.

> Sunflower oil consists of over 70 percent LA but contains almost no ALA. The same applies to safflower and corn oils. Rapeseed oil, like olive oil, contains up to 70 percent oleic acid. The remainder is a mixture of approximately 15 percent ALA and LA.

Different from all other vitamins, the F-Vitamins did not come to our attention because of a deficiency in humans, but rather through the Burrs' rat experiment. And this circumstance led to a historical error of great importance for human well-being because alone, these F-vitamins are not yet actual active ingredients. They are a few kinks short of developing their biological effect. The rats, which have contributed to the discovery of the two "F vitamins," have always been foragers throughout their evolutionary history, feeding primarily on plants and their seeds. Their metabolism must therefore be able to efficiently convert the plant precursors of ALA and LA into, respectively, bioactive substances DHA and AA.[10]

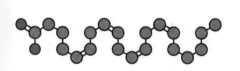

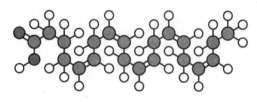

Arachidonic acid (Omega-6)   **Eicosapentaenoic acid (Omega-3)**

Left: Arachidonic acid (AA) has two kinks more than linoleic acid and is, accordingly, many times more biologically effective. Right: EPA has five kinks, two more than its precursor, ALA. Microalgae not only produce DHA, but also EPA and enrich the aquatic food chain with both bioactive omega-3 fatty acids.

To produce bioactive AA, LA is desaturated using a desaturase, creating another kink. The carbon chain is then extended by two more carbons using an elongase (the name says it all). Finally, the product is desaturated or "kinked" again using another desaturase. As a result, AA has twenty carbons in its chain, and the chain itself has four kinks, two more than the original LA—and that's exactly what makes it so biologically valuable, as we'll see.

To synthesize bioactive omega-3 fatty acids from plant ALA, our organism uses the same desaturases and the same elongase as in the production of AA from LA—albeit highly inefficiently. Eicosapentaenoic acid (EPA) is initially created from ALA. It is a bioactive omega-3 fatty acid and, like AA, has twenty carbons (*eicosa* is Greek for twenty). It has a total of five kinks (penta-en means five times unsaturated); two more than its plant precursor ALA.

EPA is an important building material for the cell membranes of all body cells, except nerve cells, where DHA is almost exclusively used. EPA is also the starting point for forming many crucial tissue hormones. Like DHA, it is a vital aquatic omega-3 fatty acid—also produced by microalgae.

Our organism can produce DHA from EPA, but extremely inefficiently. To do this, EPA is extended again twice by two carbons using the same elongases. The chain is then desaturated again, also with the same desaturase, and in a final step, the chain is shortened by two carbons. After this complicated maneuver, docosahexaenoic acid has a total of twenty-two carbons (*dosa* means twenty-two) in its carbon chain. DHA is also hexa-en, which means six times unsaturated.

In contrast to the high conversion rate in rats, these biochemical processes are extremely ineffective in humans. There is good

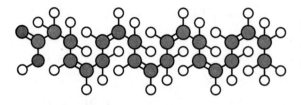

Docosahexaenoic acid (Omega-3)

DHA can be created from ALA or EPA in a complex biochemical process. This omega-3 fatty acid has twenty-two carbons and a total of six kinks.

reason for this, because our ancestors—unlike rats—were not just gatherers, but very longtime fishermen. Fish and seafood are rich in EPA and DHA. Therefore, our genetic material adapted to a basic supply of these bioactive aquatic omega-3 fatty acids. As a result, our organism is dependent on a supply of these bioactive omega-3 fatty acids for life if it is to function optimally. In fact, only a small percent of plant ALA is converted to EPA and only a small proportion of this is converted to DHA—if any. In a study on humans, a conversion rate of ALA into EPA was found to be around 7 percent[11], and in another study it was only 0.3 percent.[12] However, both studies showed almost no further conversion of EPA into DHA. Even high amounts of about one ounce (30 grams) of pure flaxseed oil per day did not lead to a measurable increase in DHA, despite the very high intake of ALA.[13] A purely vegan diet does not guarantee an adequate supply of these aquatic fatty acids—no matter how much ALA or omega-3-rich vegetable oil we consume. This means that what is essential for us is not a supply of the plant-based omega-3 fatty acid ALA, but rather a sufficient supply of the omega-3 fatty acids EPA and, above all, DHA.[14] Since these two bioactive omega-3 fatty acids are fatty acids primarily found in fish and seafood (or in oil from microalgae), I refer to them as aquatic omega-3 fatty acids to distinguish them from the terrestrial (land plants) omega-3 fatty acid, ALA.

A distinction must be made regarding the omega-3 fatty acid ALA, which occurs terrestrially (in land plants). Although we can hardly convert ALA into bioactive EPA and DHA, many doctors and alternative practitioners still often recommend flaxseed or linseed oil, which has the highest ALA concentration of all plant oils, to correct or prevent an omega-3 deficiency. There is an urgent need to rethink this. In my opinion, products should not be advertised with reference to omega-3 fatty acids if it is not clearly stated whether they are actually aquatic and, ergo, bioactive active ingredients. Otherwise, the messaging to consumers wrongly implies that these products provide them with adequate intake. The problem of inadequate endogenous EPA, and, especially, DHA production, is further exacerbated by the modern Western diet. The same desaturases and elongases are used to convert LA to AA as are used to convert ALA to EPA, and, in turn, EPA to DHA.[15] As a result, the omega-6 fatty acid LA and the omega-3 fatty acid ALA compete for the same tool to produce bioactive active ingredients—whereby LA wins due to our past as fishermen and gatherers, in which it was not EPA and DHA, but rather animal AA that was in short supply.[16] The problem is that our current diet mainly includes vegetable oils extremely rich in LA but with virtually no ALA: e.g., sunflower, corn germ, safflower, and, last but not least, soybean oil.[17] The proportion of soybean oil alone in US fast food consumption, for example, has increased by more than a thousand-fold since around the middle of the last century.[18] Soybean oil consists of around 60 percent LA and now accounts for about 7 percent of the total US food energy intake. For many years, scientists have warned about the consequences of a massive increase in LA at the expense of ALA, which within just a few decades has become the standard in all industrialized nations and, now, also in the so-called emerging countries.[19] Instead of being balanced, intake is well over ten to one favoring LA over ALA.[20]

Since the overall production rate for bioactive fatty acids from plant precursors is limited,[21] this huge increase in LA in our diet automatically means less EPA that can be produced from ALA.[22] In order to maximize the already low EPA production capacity, LA total energy intake would have to be less than 2.5 percent. But it is over 8 percent—and there is no trend reversal in sight.

As a result, there is an increasingly serious disproportion of AA and EPA (as well as DHA). And this has equally grave consequences: As early as 1997, Japanese researchers pointed out that an "omega-3 deficiency syndrome" had developed due to changes in their traditional lifestyle:[23] Reduced fish and seafood consumption, more LA-rich vegetable oils and AA-rich meat products. This is accompanied by an increased risk of previously Western forms of cancer, cardiovascular diseases, and allergies. The increase in the rate of Alzheimer's disease by a factor of seven is also explained by this change to a diet rich in omega-6 while at the same time low in omega-3.[24]

This dietary imbalance also changes human behavior. For example, a recent scientific study found that a high proportion of LA to ALA in the mother's diet negatively influences both her child's mental and psychomotor development.[25] DHA deficiency has also shown to lead to frontal lobe weakness with tendencies towards antisocial behavior (more on this on pages 75 to 90). This development has enormous negative consequences for humanity's future, which I will discuss at the end of this book. It is therefore highly recommended that these LA-rich oils be totally avoided.

THE YIN AND YANG OF
ESSENTIAL FATTY ACIDS

The omega-6 fatty acid AA is just as vital as the two omega-3 fatty acids EPA and DHA. None of these should be limited if our mental and physical potential is to fully develop and be maintained long term. However, the ratio of the two classes of fatty acids must be balanced. This is because bioactive fatty acids EPA and DHA, and AA on the other hand, are the basis for forming entire armadas of very potent tissue hormones, which have opposite effects in almost all organ systems—and work together in exactly this way to benefit our health.

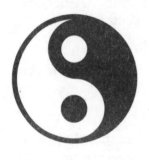

In Chinese philosophy, yin and yang stand for forces that are opposite to one another, but nevertheless related to each other and thus work together. This image also makes it easy to understand how biological processes ensure growth and stability or health.

This can best be explained by the Yin/Yang principle. This is not meant to be philosophical nor esoteric. Instead, it has a very practical and scientifically real dimension. This principle can also be found in almost all biological systems.

For example, our joints can be both bent and extended. Muscles on one side of the joint work in one direction, those on the other in the opposite. Only when both work together can we stand upright or reach for something with our hands.

Similarly, the balanced action of hormonal counterparts, which our organism synthesizes from the bioactive omega-3 and omega-6 fatty acids, stabilizes almost all biological processes in our entire organism.

The hormonal active substances formed from EPA and AA are called eicosanoids. As the name suggests, like EPA and AA themselves, they consist of twenty carbons each. There are so many eicosanoids that they are divided into different classes: prostaglandins, prostacyclins, thromboxanes, leukotrienes, or endocannabinoids. They play an important role in regulating the cardiovascular system, blood clotting, the immune system, and pain sensation. The endocannabinoids alone (via whose receptors cannabis carries out its effect) influence a wide range of biological systems: immune regulation, metabolism and energy turnover, but also sleep behavior, mood, memory, and many more.[26]

Very often the omega-3 eicosanoids, which are formed from EPA, are referred to as "good," while the omega-6 eicosanoids, which are formed from AA, are referred to as "bad." But this distinction is wrong because we need both classes. The only bad thing is the ratio because it is now completely unbalanced due to our non-germane diet: too much AA and too little EPA creates an overall harmful effect. To stay with the previous example, this is rather like only working our hamstrings and hardly ever our leg extensors. We would simply fall over or be unable to stand up at all.

Here are two important examples of the yin/yang principle of omega-6/omega-3 interaction:

- Together, the active ingredients of both classes of fatty acids regulate blood clotting. They act as opponents. When we get injured, eicosanoids produced from AA are activated first. They stimulate blood clotting and protect us from bleeding. Once bleeding has stopped, eicosanoids formed from EPA inhibit further blood clotting, which prevents an excessive and persistent tendency to clot that could lead to dangerous thrombosis, i.e., blockages of blood vessels, and, from these, blood clots could develop. Fatal heart attacks, pulmonary embolisms, and strokes would be possible consequences.

- Both classes of fatty acids are also vital in controlling the immune system. Without AA eicosanoids it would not be efficiently activated when we have an infection. EPA eicosanoids, in turn, help stop the inflammatory reaction as soon as the infection has been overcome.[27] A lack of AA would leave us defenseless against pathogens; conversely, an EPA deficiency would turn an acute inflammatory reaction into a chronic one, making us permanently ill.

As seen in the figure below, DHA is also used to produce hormonal agents. These fall under the term docosanoids because, like DHA itself, they consist of twenty-two carbons. Like EPA eicosanoids, they play an important role in stopping bleeding or an inflammatory reaction, especially in the subsequent repair of the resulting tissue damage.[28] The DHA active ingredients are therefore also referred to as protectins and as resolvins, or as a maresine (from *ma*crophage mediator in *res*olving *in*flammation). The latter group of active ingredients activates macrophages (which, as the name suggests, are "large phagocytes" that are part of our immune system). After being activated by maresins, they recognize damaged tissue, eat, and digest it.[29] In doing so, they help to

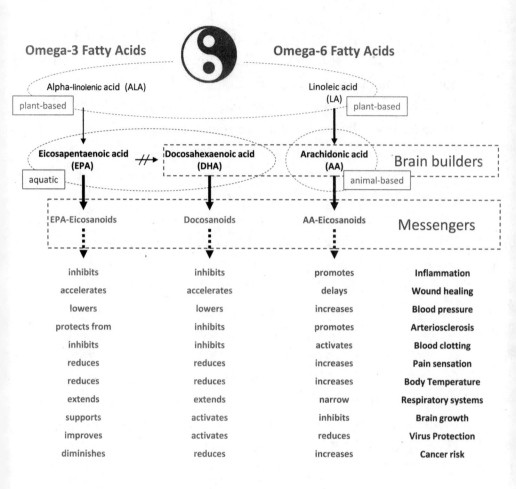

The yin and yang of omega-3 and omega-6 fatty acids. The conversion rate of plant ALA into EPA is low in humans; DHA is almost not formed at all. EPA and DHA are the essential fatty acids that we must obtain from aquatic food sources. LA can be found in abundance in almost all plant-based foods, so that enough AA can be produced from it. DHA and AA are important brain-building blocks. Absolute nutritional deficiency impairs brain growth and mental fitness maintenance. The effect of the messengers that our organism synthesizes from aquatic omega-3 fatty acids EPA and DHA, and from the animal omega-6 fatty acid AA, is oppositional in almost all biological processes.

end the disease process and, simultaneously, initiate wound healing. Docosanoids also prevent allergic reactions and reduce nerve pain resulting from tissue damage.

The formation of new nerve cells (neurogenesis) is also influenced in opposite ways by active ingredients of both fatty acid families:[30] AA eicosanoids inhibit neurogenesis, whereas DHA active ingredients activate neurogenesis (see also pages 11 to 12). Conversely, AA eicosanoids promote the breakdown of damaged nerve cells (neurodegeneration) whereas DHA blocks this process. AA is therefore considered (but only because we consume too much of it) to be a causal risk factor for preventable mental decline in old age.[31] Neuroprotectin 1 from DHA protects neurons and has exactly the opposite effect.[32]

As indicated in the previous figure, the list of the complementary functions of active substances that our organism produces from the two classes of fatty acids could be continued almost endlessly. But these few examples show what the importance of these tissue hormones is, in which areas, and what adverse health effects can be expected from a chronic nutritional imbalance.[33] We will discuss the consequences of this in detail in the next chapter, because the modern Western diet is far from having a good omega-6/3 ratio.

FATTY ACID ANALYSIS—A DROP OF BLOOD IS ENOUGH

Essential fatty acids are mainly stored in our cell membranes, where they also unfold a significant part of their biological effect. It then makes sense to determine their composition in the cell membranes. Red blood cells are best suited for fatty acid analysis. Their fatty acid composition corresponds more or less to that of all body cells,[34] and they are easy to access. Even a small drop of blood is enough to examine and calculate several important aspects of nutrition easily and relatively inexpensively. These include, among other things, the omega-6/3 quotient, the omega-3 index, cell membrane fluidity, and the percentage of harmful trans fatty acids.[35]

OMEGA-6/3 RATIO (O-6/3 R)

This value provides information about whether there's a mismatch between omega-6 fatty acid AA and omega-3 fatty acid EPA in the diet.

A ratio of less than 2.5 to 1 (omega-6 to omega-3) is ideal. If it's significantly higher, two measures must be taken: first, avoiding rich omega-6 fatty acid sources like prepared foods, meat, and sausage products as well as LA-rich oils. Second, increase intake of aquatic omega-3 fatty acids.

OMEGA-3 INDEX

The omega-3 index corresponds to the percentage of EPA and DHA in the total red blood cell membrane fatty acids and is of immense clinical importance. For example, an omega-3 index of less than 4 percent (which is unfortunately common in many Western nations) is associated with a tenfold increased risk compared to a value well above 8 percent (which is closer to that of a fisher-gatherer).[36]

Since all cell membranes (and also our fat deposits) form a large reservoir of fatty acids, the omega-3 index usually changes only very slowly—over weeks or months—when changing one's diet. The omega-3 index is our "omega-3 memory," which tells us whether we have consumed either too little or enough aquatic omega-3 fatty acids over a longer period of time.

FLUIDITY OF CELL MEMBRANES

Another interesting value indirectly determined by fatty acid analysis is that of the fluidity or flexibility of the cell membrane. This has enormous significance for health.

For example, red blood cells must push through narrow blood vessels (capillaries) to transport oxygen to the tissue. If the cell membranes of red blood cells and the cells that form capillaries were rigid, our blood vessels would become blocked. White blood cells, on the other hand, must travel through our organ tissues to detect and destroy bacteria and cancer cells. They do this in the fashion of amoebas, which, like microalgae, are part of plankton.

Finally, as I've already explained in detail in the previous chapter, communication between our nerve cells depends on the fluidity of the nerve cell membranes. This is also determined by the composition of the fatty acids it contains.

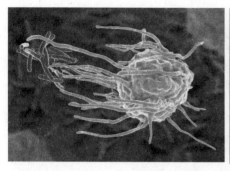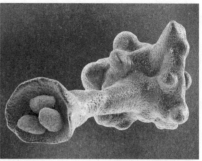

White blood cells (left) behave like amoebas (right). Both cells crawl through their surroundings and use their fluid membranes to bring bacteria inside to absorb and eat them.

A good measure of a fatty acid's ability to impart fluidity to a membrane is its melting point, which is the temperature at which it changes from a solid to a liquid. Generally, the following applies: the longer and more saturated a fatty acid, the higher the melting point and the more rigid the cell membrane. Conversely, the shorter a fatty acid is and the more kinks its carbon chain has, the lower its melting point and the higher the cell membrane's fluidity.

As shown in the following figure, the melting point increases as the number of carbons (C) increases into a chain. If it does not kink (C+0), the temperature required for liquefaction is especially high. If the somatic membranes, for example, predominantly contained the long-chain and saturated stearic acid (18C+0), they would only be fully functional at a body temperature of well over 140° Fahrenheit (60° Celsius). Coconut oil's composition from mainly medium-long fatty acids explains why it is spreadable at room temperature.

But even a single kink that turns stearic acid (18C+0) into oleic acid (18C+1) lowers the melting temperature from 156° to 60° Fahrenheit (69° to 16° Celsius). This is why olive oil is liquid

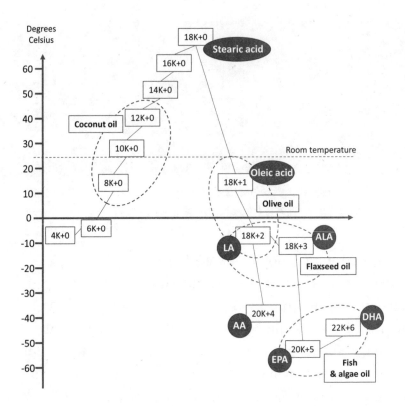

Melting temperature of fatty acids depends on chain length and the number of unsaturated carbon pairs: The shorter the carbon chain is, but the more kinks it has, the more liquid the oil that predominantly contains it.

at room temperature. As it gives our cells a high level of fluidity even at normal body temperature, oleic acid is increasingly incorporated into the maturing brain.[37]

With around 15 percent LA (18C+2) and around 70 percent ALA (18C+3), flaxseed oil consists almost exclusively of polyunsaturated fatty acids. That's why flaxseed oil is still liquid, even refrigerated. The melting point of fatty acids decreases even further when they have even more kinks. That of AA (20C+4) is significantly lower than of LA (18C+2), and the two aquatic omega-3 fatty acids EPA (20C+5) and DHA (22C+6) are still liquid even in extreme cold.

The fact that aquatic fatty acids EPA and DHA are still liquid even at cold temperatures is the reason fish store many of these fatty acids in their tissues. This is especially true for fish in polar seas. If they stored predominantly saturated fatty acids, like land animals such as pigs and cows, they would solidify in cold seawater. The different fatty acid melting temperatures allow our body cells to regulate cell membrane fluidity via their composition. A ratio of about one to one of polyunsaturated to saturated fatty acids is considered beneficial: the membranes are fluid, allowing the cells to move well without losing necessary firmness.

Fish from cold mountain streams, such as trout or brook char, are very rich in aquatic omega-3 fatty acids, with levels reaching up to 3 percent of their weight.

TRANS FATTY ACIDS

Unlike saturated fatty acids, unsaturated fatty acids are chemically unstable—the more unsaturated, the more unstable. For example, one of the two hydrogens in an unsaturated carbon pair can rearrange itself from one side to the other. It is then no longer in the cis position, like with all of our naturally "kinked" unsaturated fatty acids, but in a so-called trans position, because the two hydrogens are opposite each other. This means that a cis-fatty acid becomes a trans-fatty acid, as can be seen in the following figure, using the example of trans-oleic acid. Although still unsaturated, the rearrangement causes it to lose its kink and stretch (compare to cis-oleic acid on page 39).

This stretching causes a trans fatty acid to behave like a saturated one, although it's unsaturated: melting requires a higher temperature. Cis-oleic acid melts at 60° Fahrenheit (16 ° Celsius),

Alpha   **Omega**

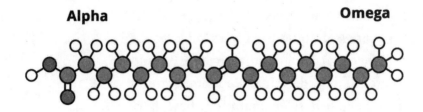

Elaidic acid (trans-D9)

Although trans fatty acids are unsaturated (see double bond between the ninth and tenth carbons), they are still stretched like a saturated fatty acid.

whereas trans-oleic acid melts at 115° Fahrenheit (46.5° Celsius). Easy to imagine what happens if too many trans fatty acids are consumed due to a poor diet, and incorporated into cell membranes, instead of cis fatty acids: fluidity decreases.

Unfortunately, this "oversight" is the rule because, as already mentioned, trans fatty acids are unsaturated despite their stretching, and, like cis fatty acids, are preferentially incorporated into cell membranes. The resulting reduced fluidity disrupts communication between cells and important processes within the cell membrane. Red blood cells, which are less fluid, make blood flow more difficult, increasing the risk of arteriosclerosis. The immune system is disrupted, heightening the risk of cancer, among other things. Chronic inflammation is also one of many consequences of a high intake of trans fatty acids.

Trans fatty acids are formed during frying with cooking oils that are rich in polyunsaturated fatty acids.[38]

A team of researchers from Harvard University summarized some of the health-threatening effects of trans fatty acids.[39] Their findings are based on well-controlled clinical and epidemiological studies as well as countless laboratory tests. Trans fatty acids increase the risk of Alzheimer's disease and Type 2 diabetes. They worsen cholesterol metabolism and increase the risk of vascular dementia. That is why trans fatty acids are extremely unhealthy for us even in small amounts. A daily intake of just one teaspoon (five grams) of trans fatty acids doubles the risk of coronary heart disease (angina and heart attack), which is why you should stay well below this level. It's not even clear whether there is an amount of intake that could be described as harmless.

Trans fatty acids are formed when deep-frying or frying using cooking oils rich in cis-polyunsaturated fatty acids. These include sunflower, corn germ, safflower, or rapeseed oil. As such, none of these oils should be heated.

Trans fatty acids are also a byproduct of hardening vegetable oils. By intentionally stretching the cis fatty acids it contains, an oil that is liquid at room temperature becomes solid and spreadable—but also unhealthy. Trans fatty acids are often found in convenience foods, chips, and cookies.

Trans fatty acids are also produced by bacterial processes in ruminants' (e.g., goats, sheep, cows) rumens. They are found in concentrations of 4 to 6 percent in the fat of dairy products and animal fatty tissue. However, values of 10 percent have also been measured when the animals are fed food rich in cis fatty acids.[40]

As early as the end of the 1970s, the World Health Organization (WHO) called on its member countries to ban the use of trans fatty acids. But so far little has been done to protect consumers and WHO warnings have not resulted in laws that actually protect us consumers. On the contrary. In Europe, lawmakers are particularly industry-friendly and have even legally banned labelling trans fatty acids on packaging.[41] Thus, anyone who does not put trans fatty acids in their processed food lacks a competitive advantage—rather, the system favors those who do and thereby endanger our health. Politics always follows the recommendations of the most powerful voices in the food industry.

A fatty acid analysis is also recommended to check your diet and not be surprised by hidden trans fatty acids. The best thing you can do for your health is to cook for yourself. My own test results, based on the principles of a diet I set out in my book, *Kopfküche*,[42] were well within the range of normal:

Omega-6/Omega-3 ratio	2.5 to 1
Omega-3 index	11 percent
Fluidity of cell membranes	1.07
Trans fatty acids	0.14 percent

TOXIC SUBSTANCES FROM UNSATURATED FATTY ACIDS

The development of harmful trans fatty acids is not the only problem, which is why we should treat oils rich in unsaturated fatty acids with caution. Unsaturated fatty acids also like to react with oxygen. This creates so-called oxygen radicals. These are toxic, highly reactive chemicals that should not be in your food. These radicals catalyze several chemical reactions, all of which have a characteristic result: the oil becomes rancid. The smell is consequently extremely unpleasant and thus fulfills an important biological purpose: it warns us of spoiled food.

When sunflower oil is heated, the omega-6 fatty acids it contains oxidize to produce the highly toxic aldehyde 4-hydroxynonenal (4-HNE), whose effect promotes, for example, Alzheimer's, Parkinson's and many other serious brain diseases.[43]

There is, of course, a risk of forming trans fatty acids, oxygen radicals and toxins such as 4-HNE, when heating any oils that are particularly rich in polyunsaturated fatty acids. Due to the laws of chemistry, all these unhealthy changes occur several times faster at high temperatures than at room temperature or in the refrigerator. Light can also cause these changes. To prevent toxins from forming, oils rich in unsaturated fatty acids should

Fish should not have an unpleasant smell. If it does, the rancid odor is a warning sign that the aquatic omega-3 fatty acids have oxidized, making both the fish and the fatty acids inedible.

be kept in dark bottles and stored in the refrigerator. This is particularly true for fish, krill, and algae oil, as the aquatic omega-3 fatty acids they contain have the most unsaturated kinks and are therefore extremely susceptible to transforming into trans fatty acids.

Compared to sunflower, corn germ, safflower, rapeseed, or linseed oil, which mainly consist of polyunsaturated fatty acids, olive oil contains over 70 percent monounsaturated oleic acid. It is thus less sensitive. However, it should not be fried too hot (not above the smoke point of about 356° Fahrenheit (180° Celsius). Coconut oil, however, can practically not form any trans fats or oxygen radicals because it consists primarily of saturated fatty acids, and is therefore ideally suited for roasting and baking.

* * *

You now know that polyunsaturated omega-3 and omega-6 fatty acids are essential. You also now know that a balanced ratio is important and that we are subject to a historical error when it comes to omega-3 fatty acid food sources. Contrary to popular opinion, we must rely on aquatic foods; only these contain sufficient EPA and DHA. ALA is just a precursor of these two bioactive fatty acids. Our organism can barely produce EPA and DHA from plant-based ALA-rich oil, like from flaxseed. ALA-rich vegetable oils are still healthy because they contain little LA and, therefore, counteract an oversupply of this omega-6 fatty acid. Olive oil is also used for this purpose, though it hardly contains any ALA. Therefore, if you replace sunflower oil with olive oil, you reduce your LA intake sixfold.

The need to reduce LA, and especially AA-rich foods and to increase the consumption of aquatic omega-3 fatty acids in the modern Western diet has been known in scientific circles at least since mid-last century.[44] Nevertheless, irrational development continued. If we add trans fatty acids and toxic oxidation products such as HNE to this unhealthy mix, then we have a good explanation for countless widespread diseases and over 90 percent of all deaths that are now normal in industrialized nations—even though these are all unnatural, and thus avoidable.

PART III

PANDEMICS DUE TO AQUATIC OMEGA-3 DEFICIENCY

MENTAL DEVELOPMENTAL DISORDERS

For to everyone who has, more will be given, and he will have abundance; but from him who does not have, even what he has will be taken away.

—*Gospel According to Matthew 25:29*

THE BREAST MILK QUALITY FACTOR

The human brain experiences its greatest growth spurt in the last trimester of pregnancy and the first year-and-a-half of life. Its weight increases from less than a quarter pound (100 grams) to almost two and a half pounds (1100 grams), an eleven-fold increase.[1] The total amount of DHA that the growing brain incorporates into its cell membranes increases thirty-five-fold, i.e., disproportionately.[2] Even without accounting for DHA's many other functions (as well as those of EPA) as a hormone-like growth and protective factor for the brain, which we discussed in detail earlier, this ratio makes it clear why a lack of aquatic omega-3 fatty acids limits brain growth.

Neither the unborn child nor the infant can synthesize DHA from plant ALA.[3] For this reason, an adequate supply of DHA is so important in this phase, which is crucial for the development of mental abilities.[4] The child obtains DHA (and EPA) through the placenta before birth, and after via breast milk.[5] Baby formula

The mental health of the child depends on the DHA content in breast milk, and this, in turn, depends on the mother's adequate intake.

enriched with aquatic omega-3 fatty acids would be an adequate alternative if necessary. One study showed no difference in the development of visual acuity and intelligence as compared to breastfeeding.[6]

In order to provide the growing child's brain with DHA and EPA, the mother has three natural sources available:

- Internal production from plant-based ALA
- Stored aquatic omega-3 fatty acids
- Nutrition supplemented with aquatic omega-3 fatty acids during pregnancy and breastfeeding

Let's consider each of these sources.

Internal Production

It has been reported that women of childbearing age can produce some DHA from ALA, unlike men of the same age.[7] However, internal production seems to be an insufficient emergency mechanism because, according to the results of another study, taking in ALA-rich flaxseed oil does not lead to an increase in DHA in the blood to supply the growing child via the placenta or in breast milk after birth—contrasted with the EPA concentration in blood and breast milk.[8]

Even a dietary supplement with ready-made EPA does not increase DHA concentration.[9] It is therefore important that the mother take in ready-made DHA from aquatic sources if the child is not to suffer a serious deficiency. If she is unable to breastfeed, the newborn needs formula enriched with aquatic omega-3 fatty acids.[10]

Storage

Children adequately supplied with DHA have the best chance of optimal brain development. In the Paleolithic period, this increased the probability of reaching adulthood to pass on one's own genetic material to the next generation. A good DHA supply therefore has a cross-generational effect and acts as a driver of evolutionary optimization. From an evolutionary biology perspective, it makes perfect sense that women especially developed the ability to store aquatic omega-3 fatty acids in their fatty tissue. This had the advantage that an expectant mother could use the previously created deposits to protect herself or her unborn child, even when she may not have sufficient access to marine sources of these essential fatty acids during the child's crucial brain growth phase to provide her infant with DHA.

The female storage location for polyunsaturated fatty acids is the fatty tissue in the hips and thighs, but not the waist. The waist is where saturated fatty acids are primarily stored, long-term, in both sexes.[11] The fact that the risk of mental maldevelopment due to a lack of DHA is far greater than due to an energy deficit could explain the global and culturally-independent male preference for a woman with a wasp waist body type—little belly fat, but more hip fat.[12] In other words, men could be genetically unconsciously programmed to prefer women with a correspondingly lower waist/hip ratio (WHR), of about 0.7 to benefit their potential offspring.

A smaller WHR is actually associated with a higher DHA concentration in both the mother's blood and milk, whereas the opposite was measured in women with larger WHR:[13] lower DHA and higher AA concentrations. It is therefore not surprising that a study of around two thousand mother/child pairs showed that the

A low waist-to-hip ratio of about 0.7 has always been considered attractive in every culture. This form of female fat distribution is associated with good DHA storage and the best developmental prospects for offspring.

mother's WHR was inversely related to the development of her child's mental performance: with a WHR below 0.72, the children showed the best test results in terms of intellectual fitness, while with a WHR above 0.92, the children showed the worst results.[14] The same also applied to the women themselves. Their mental performance increased as their WHR of over 0.92 approached 0.72.

The fact that mothers care for their children through their hip deposits during pregnancy and breastfeeding is also reflected in the fact that those deposits become smaller with each pregnancy. As a result, WHR increases from birth to birth.[15] This also applies to women in traditional foraging societies who do not live in energy surplus like those in industrialized nations (which causes WHR as belly fat and waist size increase), as found in another study.[16] Evidence was also provided that a lower WHR is a good indicator of a woman's health and increases her chance of having many offspring.

Based on these findings, it is recommended that women fill their deposits with aquatic omega-3 fatty acids long before becoming pregnant—for the health of their future children and their own.[17]

Nutrition

A worldwide study found that DHA concentration in breast milk varies greatly. It is always highest where women live near the coast or where a lot of fish and seafood are traditionally consumed and is very low when women avoid these foods.[18] In contrast, the AA concentration hardly shows any major fluctuations. It is largely stable, regardless of diet type. This is because, as a rule, no diet leads to a deficiency in this omega-6 fatty acid. Even with a diet low in AA, a sufficiently large proportion of the amount of AA in breast milk still comes from the mother's stores.[19]

On the other hand, if there is a fundamentally deficient supply of aquatic omega-3 fatty acids, almost no corresponding deposits are created. As a result, an adequate supply of these essential fatty acids to the child during pregnancy and breastfeeding is particularly dependent on the mother's diet.

> The diet of the expectant mother has a decisive influence on her child's mental, social, and emotional abilities.

FROM MATERNAL OMEGA-3 INDEX TO A CHILD'S IQ

A maternal diet rich in aquatic omega-3 fatty acids results in a good omega-3 index. The amount of DHA supplied during pregnancy is directly related to the amount that reaches the fetus. With a limited intake of omega-6 fatty acids, the omega-6/3 ratio (O-6/3-Q) is optimized. Both have a direct influence on the development of the child's mental performance:

- The more fish the mother consumes in the crucial growth phases of the child's brain, the better the child's mental development progresses.[20] A daily half-tablespoon of DHA-rich cod liver oil during pregnancy and breastfeeding resulted in an on average 4 percent higher mental fitness at birth, compared to the children of mothers who only consumed corn oil.[21]
- The higher the intake in the mother, the better the child's hand-eye coordination. This effect is visible even two and a half years after birth.[22]

- Head circumference and birth weight of first-born children to women who consumed DHA, e.g., in the form of algae oil, are larger than of those who consumed it hardly or not at all.[23] A larger head circumference at birth tends to go hand in hand with the improved development of the child's intelligence.[24]
- In Inuit children, a direct relationship could be demonstrated between the DHA concentration in the umbilical cord—as a measure of the prenatal supply of this brain-building material to the developing child—and mental performance and memory capacity, even eleven years after birth.[25]

According to mathematical calculations based on a whole series of results from such studies and investigations, the following relationship results: for approximately every quarter teaspoon (one gram) of DHA that the mother consumes daily during this important phase of development for the child, the child's intelligence quotient (IQ) increases between 0.8 to 1.8 points.[26]

Since a human diet rich in DHA is seen as a "species-appropriate" norm from an evolutionary biology perspective, in my opinion, one should not speak of an increase in intelligence through aquatic omega-3 fatty acids. Rather, an unnatural lack of them leads to a loss of intelligence—and this adverse effect is enduring:

- This loss of intelligence in the child due to a maternal DHA deficiency before, during, and after delivery could still be demonstrated at the age of seven.[27]
- In another study, such a long-term effect of a corresponding lack of supply was still clearly visible even fifteen years after birth. In the countries with the best omega-6/3 ratio

in breast milk (Japan, Korea, and Singapore), children performed best in the so-called PISA study.[28] High DHA levels were accompanied by good school performance. However, high LA levels, which are typical of the modern Western diet with correspondingly high amounts of LA-rich oils, significantly worsened the chances of doing well in school.

- When predicting future academic performance, O-6/3-Q in breast milk is a more accurate and clear-cut prognostic factor than per capita income, per-child government spending on schooling, or any other measure studied to date.

That should give us pause. In my opinion, there is hardly more compelling evidence of the importance of early childhood brain development for our long-term well-being, nor any clearer evidence of the role that maternal nutrition plays in this. These results also show it is worth investing in an adequate supply of aquatic omega-3 fatty acids instead of just investing in the education system.

AQUATIC FATTY ACIDS PREVENT PREMATURE BIRTHS

A premature birth is, by definition, a birth before the thirty-eighth week of pregnancy. Around 15 million children worldwide are born prematurely every year, of which over a million die from the associated complications.[29] Most premature births occur in the poor regions of the world, but the rate is also quite high in rich industrialized nations. For example, in the United States, one in eight pregnancies results in a premature birth, with all the health disadvantages for the child.

Every week that a child is born prematurely reduces its chance of receiving the supply of aquatic omega-3 fatty acids necessary for this phase of development. All infants born before the fortieth week of pregnancy, therefore, suffer from a DHA deficiency.[30]

However, the shorter the pregnancy, the greater the undersupply of DHA (and, of course, EPA).[31] Extremely premature babies (i.e., babies born before twenty-eight weeks) receive only about a third of the amount of DHA from standard care that they would have via the uterus.[32] It is therefore not surprising that premature babies particularly benefit from dietary supplementation with aquatic omega-3 fatty acids.[33]

It would, of course, be best if children were not born prematurely in the first place. Unfortunately, that trend is heading in the wrong direction: In just a decade (from 1992 to 2002), for example, in the United States, the average duration of pregnancy has shortened by a whole week.[34] Here, too, the O-6/3-Q plays a role, because messenger substances derived from the omega-6 fatty acid accelerate the birth process—unlike those derived from aquatic omega-3 fatty acids.[35] According to the results of a meta-study (in which all relevant previous studies have been summarized and evaluated), the risk of premature birth is therefore reduced by a total of one-third with the intake of aquatic omega-3 fatty acids.[36] In high-risk pregnancies, the risk of premature childbirth is reduced by even more than 60 percent through an adequate supply of aquatic omega-3 fatty acids. Overall, the duration of pregnancy increases by an average of around two weeks. That's a lot, because every week the child's intellectual performance increases. In terms of IQ, this is expressed in a total of about 2.5 points.[37]

It is therefore obvious that for these reasons it is worthwhile for the expectant mother to eat a balanced diet with enough aquatic omega-3 fatty acids. Such an investment in appropriate foods even saves money, as experts have calculated.[38] According to this, the costs of nutritional supplementation with aquatic omega-3 fatty acids during pregnancy are only about a tenth of what would be expected to be spent on a lengthier hospital stay and treatments due to the consequences of a lack of aquatic omega-3 fatty acids.

> A maternal diet with aquatic omega-3 fatty acids in a balanced ratio to bioactive omega-6 fatty acids reduces the risk of premature birth, improves the newborn's mental development, and simultaneously increases its chances of survival.

THE FRONTAL LOBE—WHAT MAKES HUMANS HUMAN

We owe our dominance as a species in particular to the existence of our frontal lobe.[39] As shown in the first chapter, this brain region is also the key distinguishing feature between our brain, i.e., that of a former fisher-gatherer, and that of the Neanderthal, who was a hunter-gatherer. Since the formation of our frontal lobe was the last decisive step in our evolution, our individual development (ontogenesis) in a certain way repeats our tribal development (phylogenesis):[40] as part of early childhood brain development, it is the last brain region to experience the decisive growth spurt.

The ratio of AA to DHA in the growth of our frontal lobe reflects both quantitatively and qualitatively our prehistoric adaptation to the diet of a fisher-gatherer culture: it progresses from AA-rich to DHA-rich, as shown in the figure below.

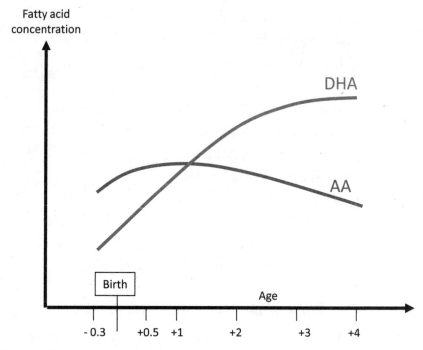

The concentration of the essential fatty acids AA and DHA in the developing frontal lobe.[41]

Until the beginning of the last trimester, the frontal lobe is still relatively rich in AA and poor in DHA.

The omega-6 to omega-3 ratio is around two. But during the subsequent growth spurt, DHA concentration approaches that of AA, only to reverse course during the first few years of life: DHA becomes the dominant essential fatty acid in the human frontal lobe. Once again: the ratio of these two fatty acids is roughly the same as that found in the diet of a fisher-gatherer.

Frontal lobe development in this phase is not only accompanied by the rapid development of new nerve cells, but also by their complex networking with other important brain regions. As a result, the frontal lobe can access all information relevant to life.

According to the latest findings, this networking is also an essential criterion for the development of human intelligence; whereby the more connected, the smarter.[42] At the same time, there is an increased isolation of the pathways (the technical term is myelination). This results in safer and faster data transmission. This optimization process 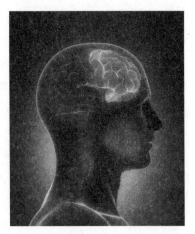 is also an essential basis for developing our emotional, social, and rational intelligence and runs at full speed between the sixth and twenty-fourth month after birth. Since the insulating material, the "myelin", consists largely of DHA, a sufficient supply of aquatic omega-3 fatty acids is required.[43]

This sensitive developmental time frame for networking and optimization, as well as the simultaneous high requirement for aquatic omega-3 fatty acids, could perhaps explain why in most traditional cultures, weaning does not take place until shortly before the end of the second year of life.[44] A nursing mother's diet based on aquatic food sources supports the development of an optimally connected and functioning frontal lobe, i.e., the seat of our executive functions and almost all higher mental activities.[45]

As I mentioned in the first chapter, the executive tasks of the frontal lobe include setting goals as well as the strategic and tactical planning to achieve them.[46] What matters is setting priorities and coordinating courses of action in a targeted manner. It also contains our short-term or working memory. The frontal lobe is crucial for conscious control of our attention and motor activity when implementing planned actions. In addition, the frontal lobe has the ability to constantly reassess the consequences of our actions and, if necessary, adapt our courses of action. Last but not least, the frontal lobe gives us both the emotional and social skills to motivate ourselves and other people, but also, if necessary, to slow down using impulse control. To do this, it uses its ability to develop language. Language allows us to coordinate optimally with others, exchange experiences, and communicate ideas.

In short, the properties of the frontal lobe form the basis of all types of human behavior and actions—including social interaction.[47]

FRONTAL LOBE DAMAGE DUE TO MALNUTRITION

If we consider the frontal lobe's versatile and unique functions, we can appreciate the serious consequences from its development being disrupted, as shown in the following figure.

The maturation of the frontal lobe occurs in phases and each phase is uniquely susceptible to disruption. Diseases such as ADHD, autism, schizophrenia, depression, and many others that we will discuss in this chapter are rightly associated with disorders in frontal lobe development and connectivity. Drugs like as alcohol, nicotine, and many others are known to cause such mental developmental disorders, psychological disorders, and illnesses.

While the consumption of such toxins and their problematic consequences dominate the media, the much more common causes of impaired frontal lobe development are mostly ignored: a lack of supply of essential nutritional components to the developing brain. These include, in particular, the aquatic omega-3 fatty acids as the global undersupply poses a particular problem

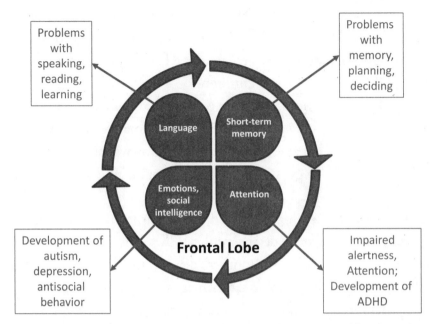

Disruptions to the frontal lobe's development are accompanied by a loss of function and increased risk of mental disorders.

because it cannot be solved with conventional nutritional strategies (see next chapter). I will, therefore, focus on this deficiency and its consequences for individual and global development. However, deficiencies in other essential nutritional components have equally serious consequences.

Children who were undersupplied with aquatic omega-3 fatty acids because their mothers did not consume enough during pregnancy and lactation often show abnormalities that can be traced back to delayed and disrupted development of the frontal lobe:

- Infants who suffer from a deficiency in essential omega-3 fatty acids are less able to deal with even harmless changes in their environment and are more restless.[48]

- As fourteen-month-old toddlers, they show significantly reduced word production and word comprehension.[49]
- Another study revealed a reduced attention span and easy distraction of these children.[50]
- Even for school age, memory retention was poorer.[51]
- At the age of eight, suboptimal performance in the areas of prosocial behavior and communication was also noted.[52] In addition, linguistic intelligence remains underdeveloped.

A child's mental development, and thus, their future opportunities depend to a large extent on the mother's diet. This is not negotiable. However, all is not lost if the mother's diet isn't optimal, because even after weaning, a diet with aquatic omega-3 fatty acids continues to be crucial for the further development of mental performance:

- Dietary supplementation with DHA leads to increased frontal lobe activity in healthy children and young adults, especially during exercises requiring increased attention.[53] This could be measured using imaging techniques.
- A further study showed that in the second phase of increased frontal lobe connectivity (between the ages of seven and nine years), any reading difficulties that may be present can be improved by administering DHA.[54] The leaders of the corresponding study summarized their results as follows: "DHA supplementation appears to offer a safe and effective way to improve reading and behavior in healthy but poorly performing children from mainstream schools."
- Conversely, schoolchildren's existing reading ability progressively deteriorates if they do not consume any aquatic omega-3 fatty acids, as compared to their schoolmates.[55]

- More than half of eight- to twelve-year-old schoolchildren who received a dietary supplement with aquatic omega-3 fatty acids as part of another study were able to concentrate better and were more receptive. After just three months, an average improvement of 70 percent was achieved.[56]

Equally impressive is the result of another work that seems to bring all of these results to a common denominator: Schoolchildren between the ages of nine and eleven who ate fish at least once a week scored about five points higher in intelligence in almost all test areas than those who never or very rarely ate fish.[57]

If you also take into account the corresponding intelligence-inhibiting effects caused by a lack of aquatic omega-3 fatty acids in early childhood, this single nutritional measure alone causes a difference of over ten IQ points. In addition, there are enormous effects on the development of social and emotional intelligence as well as many other frontal lobe functions.

Due to the diverse neurobiological functions of aquatic omega-3 fatty acids, many experts are convinced that both an absolute and a relative deficiency of these fatty acids in relation to the inflammatory omega-6 fatty acids (i.e., a disrupted omega-6/3-quotient) is partly responsible for a wide spectrum of neuro-psychiatric developmental disorders.[58] These include, as I said, ADHD, autism, schizophrenia, and depression, which I will discuss later, as well as other mental illnesses such as borderline personality disorder, which would go beyond the scope of this book to discuss. All those affected are usually diagnosed with a deficiency in aquatic omega-3 fatty acids.[59]

THE AD(H)D PARADOX

In more and more children, frontal lobe development is slowing down. A major reason for this is our modern diet, which presents with a lack of aquatic omega-3 fatty acids and many other deficits in essential micronutrients, along with a lifestyle that is generally no longer species-appropriate (e.g., lack of sleep and exercise). This leads to an absolute delay in development, including school readiness.

At the same time, our modern, performance-oriented society is constantly accelerating the norm of when a child is considered ready for school; children start school earlier and earlier. Society demands that our children adapt to the modern adult lifestyle at an ever earlier age (getting up early, sitting still for long periods of time, acquiring abstract knowledge, etc.). However, this only works when the frontal lobe is already at an advanced stage. But if social expectations become more and more urgent and frontal lobe development is simultaneously delayed, then the disproportion between the two grows. As a result, fewer and fewer children can keep up with this trend from a species-appropriate childhood to an economically compliant childhood. This cultural development, which slows down children's brain development and at the same time expects accelerated brain maturation, explains the AD(H)D paradox.

The result of this opposite development is an absolute and relative attention deficit (AD) in our children, often combined with a hyperactivity disorder (HD). Parents and teachers suffer from this homemade AD(H)D paradox—but above all, the children are affected. The disease-defining symptoms include:

- Problems with attention or concentration on a given topic
- Immature impulse control

- Hyperactivity that manifests itself in physical restlessness

> ADHD is a disorder of frontal brain maturation, both in absolute terms and relative to the excessive expectations of a performance-driven industrial society.

Hyperactivity (lack of self-control) is not always present, which is why the (H) is in parentheses.

Strangely enough, genetic causes have repeatedly been enlisted to explain what is now the most common "childhood disease."[60] This reassures the parents (you haven't done anything wrong) and the treating doctors (only medication helps, you can help via the prescription pad). But the enormous frequency of AD(H)D occurring in over 5 percent of all children (the unreported cases is probably significantly higher) clearly speaks against a genetic cause. On one hand, no genetic change (mutation) can develop as quickly as AD(H)D to reach pandemic proportions. On the other hand, in my opinion, there's no plausible evolutionary advantage for such a developmental delay in frontal lobe development that would explain such an effective selection of such a hypothetical mutation.

In keeping with the idea of a genetic cause is the widespread belief that qualitative deviations from the expectations defined by industrial society can only be corrected with the help of industrial products, i.e., medication. This makes the ADHD paradox an ADHD irony. Most stimulant medications only serve to mask the symptoms of a relative development delay. However, this does not eliminate the symptoms' causes, resulting in further postponement of absolute frontal lobe maturation, and there's a risk that the developmental delay will turn into a chronic developmental disorder that can last into adulthood—which actually happens in over half of the cases.[61]

However, our genetic makeup is important in explaining ADHD because it tells us quite precisely what a species-appropriate child development entails. Since our social norms do not account for essential aspects, the only logical explanation for the pandemic occurrence of AD(H)D is the increasing discrepancy between "species-appropriate" and "economically compliant." The frequent side effects of AD(H)D are also the result of delayed frontal lobe development. These include:

- Problems with reading and spelling.[62] Almost half of children with ADHD have an associated developmental disorder.
- Depression.[63] It is five times more common in AD(H)D patients than in children and adolescents without this diagnosis.[64] Up to 50 percent develop a depressive mood, usually several years after the onset of AD(H)D. This is considered an emotional, stress-related consequence of the AD(H)D problem. As I will show, however, the underlying tendency to develop depression is based on a growth disorder of emotional memory (see pages 90 to 95). This usually has the same causes as the disrupted frontal lobe maturation.
- Anxiety disorders.[65] About a quarter of children diagnosed with AD(H)D suffer from anxiety related to failure.
- A not yet fully developed working memory.[66] This leads especially to problems with spoken instructions. On the other hand, play instructions are largely remembered, understood, and implemented without any problems— typical for children, one might almost say.

- Sleep disorders.[67] These are frequent and exacerbate the overall problem, because sleep is of enormous importance for frontal lobe development and functioning. There is now good evidence that an improvement in sleep quality can be achieved by correcting a poor supply of aquatic omega-3 fatty acids.[68]

Since dietary deficiencies are responsible for the absolute delay in frontal lobe development, correction of these nutritional deficiencies should be the primary therapeutic measure. In fact, children with AD(H)D consistently have a low omega-3 fatty acid status.[69] Due to the clear frontal lobe development disorder and the fact that this is partly caused by the lack of aquatic omega-3 fatty acids increasingly common in our modern society, in my opinion this requires a review and, as quickly as possible, a correction of the omega-3 fatty acid deficiency. For example, in children diagnosed with ADHD, who were about two years behind in the development of their frontal lobe compared to their schoolmates of the same age, a four-month intake of aquatic omega-3 fatty acids improved their reading and writing skills.[70] Their social skills and ability to concentrate also developed more quickly. Comparably positive results have now been obtained from a whole series of clinical trials, which were summarized and analyzed in a meta-study in 2017.[71] Overall, there was a clear improvement in the symptoms through aquatic omega-3 fatty acids "therapy." Correcting this deficiency enabled and accelerated the delayed or slowed frontal lobe development. I would not call the corrective measures therapy, but simply a natural, species-appropriate diet.

Accordingly, other nutritionally-related maldevelopments can also delay frontal lobe maturation. For example, there is a correlation between the risk of ADHD and the frequency of so-called junk food consumption, whereas a balanced and healthy diet represents a protective factor.[72] This includes, among other things, vitamin D.[73] Ultimately, deficiencies in vitamins and trace elements must be diagnosed and corrected in all children, and ideally even in expectant mothers.

However, one should exercise patience and not expect that an absolute developmental disorder that arose due to a chronic deficiency that lasted several years can be corrected in just a few weeks. Brain health is a lifelong task. To protect the child, one should correct not only the absolute deficiency but also the relative delay in frontal lobe development. However, this can only be achieved by reducing the demands of a performance society primarily geared towards economic and, thus, academic success. That would fundamentally be better than giving children performance-enhancing drugs.

AUTISM—PERMANENT IMMATURITY

Autism encompasses a further spectrum of frontal lobe neurological developmental disorders characterized by impairments in social interactions and communication as well as by restricted, repetitive, and stereotyped behavior patterns. In addition to these core impairment symptoms, people with autism often suffer from AD(H)D, anxiety, and sleep disorders. Autism is also to be viewed as a disorder of frontal lobe development, which usually becomes apparent around the age of three at the latest.

Curse or blessing? Due to a tendency towards comparable deficits in social interaction and behavior pattern variability, Asperger's Syndrome is considered part of the autism spectrum. I think this is wrong because there are considerable differences. In contrast to those with so-called high-functioning autism, children with Asperger's syndrome do not show any delay in language development and typically even begin to speak at an early age. They also often have special talents in rational-analytical thinking and generally have above-average intelligence. It may well be that this is not a delayed development, just a different development. Asperger's has brought us many scientific, technological, and cultural advances through the ability to perceive the world differently. Asperger's syndrome is thus an invaluable part of the human development spectrum from a socio-cultural point of view—unlike autism.[74]

Only one child in about two thousand suffered from autism in the middle of the last century. That was 0.05 percent. Today the rate is over forty children—over 2 percent.[75] No other illness of the child's mind, not even ADHD, increased so rapidly. This rapid growth in the prevalence of autistic disorders paralleled the increase in diets of omega-6-rich foods, which was accompanied by a decreased supply of high-quality omega-3 fatty acids.[76]

An excess of AA leads to a relative deficiency of DHA, even if an expectant mother were to consume enough DHA, because these two fatty acids block each other, both during transport across the placenta and after, when transported into the child's brain. An absolute lack of aquatic omega-3 fatty acids exacerbates the undersupply of the child's brain, leading to a disrupted synapse formation in the frontal lobe and impairment of its

Autism is a lifelong condition resulting from a developmental disorder of the frontal brain, with symptoms that appear in early childhood.

nerve cell connectivity—and, thus, to the well-known neuronal disorders typical of autism.[77]

Outside this early childhood time frame, correction is difficult, and the results of most omega-3 studies are, unfortunately, rather sobering.[78] Nevertheless, supplementing with omega-3 is not necessarily useless: an initial study, in which autistic children were treated with aquatic omega-3 fatty acids, showed a favorable influence on concentration, eye contact, speech development, and motor skills.[79]

SCHIZOPHRENIA AND THE OMEGA-3 EFFECT

The term schizophrenia derives from ancient Greek *schizein* for "to split or splinter" and *phren*, meaning "mind or soul." This very serious neurodegenerative (brain-destroying) disease is characterized by delusions, hallucinations, and cognitive problems. It typically begins in early adulthood.

During puberty and until the end of adolescence, up to the age of around twenty-four, a natural "re-wiring" of the frontal lobe occurs. Breaking some old connections and forming many new ones is extremely important for developing individuality as we mature into independently thinking and acting adults. This process helps the growing brain challenge acquired social norms. This vulnerable and often contentious time also promotes personality development from a cultural perspective—as long as there are no serious deficiencies in building and messenger substances, traumatic experiences, or toxins such as nicotine, caffeine, or alcohol, which have a disruptive influence.

Schizophrenia is no longer a rare disease: in the United States alone, there are 2.8 million affected individuals.

These substances, when taken during this phase of frontal lobe reorganization, are particularly serious risk factors for schizophrenia. In contrast, fish consumption has been shown to reduce the risk of developing schizophrenia.[80] Fish provides many micronutrients, almost all of which can be responsible for this protection: Vitamin A, D, almost all vitamin B variants, as well as some trace elements and, last but not least, the aquatic omega-3 fatty acids.

There should be no deficiency in any of these active ingredients during brain development if we want to fully hone our mental fitness—and none afterwards, if we do not want to lose it again. This shouldn't surprise anyone after everything that has been said so far, since after all, these are all essential. Nevertheless, aquatic omega-3 fatty acids seem to play a very special role: targeted nutritional supplementation protects schizophrenia patients from typical loss of brain mass.[81] Clinical studies have also shown that aquatic omega-3 fatty acids attenuate psychotic symptoms—without the undesirable side effects produced by standard medications.[82]

In a high-profile study, thirteen- to twenty-five-year-old patients at risk of schizophrenia were given either aquatic omega-3 fatty acids or a placebo for a short period (three months).[83] Over the next nine months, the probability of suffering another psychotic episode in the omega-3 group was almost six times lower than in the placebo group. This result was so spectacular that researchers chose to extend the observation period a further six years. Expectations were confirmed: while 40 percent of the placebo-treated subjects developed manifest schizophrenia, in the omega-3 group less than 10 percent did—and this was highly unanticipated; after all, the three-month "therapy" was, by then, several years prior.[84]

However, the result can be explained by the fact that the aquatic omega-3 fatty acids necessary in the pubertal and post-pubertal phase (up to young adulthood) to develop your own personality— one that questions societal norms—should definitely not be lacking. Even short-term correction of a deficiency in essential brain-building materials during this period of psychological development has long-term effects.[85] It would be better, in any case, not to allow a deficit to arise in the first place and to supply yourself adequately long-term.

Both general psychological symptoms and the ability to "function" in everyday life improved as compared to the placebo group: "The majority of participants from the omega-3 group had a full-time job at the end of the study period, showed no severe functional limitations and no longer experienced any psychotic symptoms," reports the study team in their scientific article, adding: "To our knowledge, this is the first evidence that treatment with omega-3 fatty acids can prevent the transition to a full-blown psychotic illness." The researchers also write that there is hope that there will be "alternatives to treatment with psychotropic drugs."

For me, however, the question is why such study results are discussed as a therapeutic option, but there's no call for fundamental preventative measures. Instead of "treating" a deficiency that causes a serious disease by supplementing it with food, it would be much more sensible to have a consistent diet with enough aquatic omega-3 fatty acids (as well as many other nutrients essential for brain development, like vitamin D)[86] so as not to let it become a disease at all.

DEPRESSION DURING PREGNANCY AND AFTER

Although depression is experienced in the frontal lobe, it is the result of impaired new nerve cell formation (neurogenesis) in the hippocampus, the center of our emotional memory.[87] It's important to know that the hippocampus can produce new nerve cells throughout life.[88] This process is called adult neurogenesis. It ensures that our brain can accumulate new experiential knowledge well into old age. As the hippocampus grows, so does psychological resilience. A high degree of resilience means that new situations or possible projects are perceived as less stressful.

Interestingly, several hormones released in the female organism during pregnancy and breastfeeding act as highly potent growth factors for adult neurogenesis. These include two pregnancy hormones, progesterone and estrogen, as well as the contraction-causing oxytocin, and none other than prolactin, which activates the mammary glands after birth.[89] The evolutionary sense and purpose of this hormonal growth regulation is, among other things, to prepare the female memory center for childbirth and the time after. The more stress-free and positive this is perceived to be and the more detailed the memories, the closer and more stable the mother-child relationship becomes.

Based on these connections, you can easily imagine why depression is more likely if essential nutritional components that are needed for hippocampal neurogenesis are missing—especially aquatic omega-3 fatty acids:[90] Impaired adult neurogenesis due to DHA deficiency causes reduced memory for emotional experiences and leads to decreased mental resilience. You are constantly stressed because even seemingly harmless daily events or projects are perceived as very stressful. Stress hormone levels are usually permanently elevated—a key feature of depression. Because stress hormones in turn affect neurogenesis in the hippocampus, the condition

> Lifelong motherly love is based on positive memories and depends on the undisturbed growth of the hippocampus during pregnancy and breastfeeding.

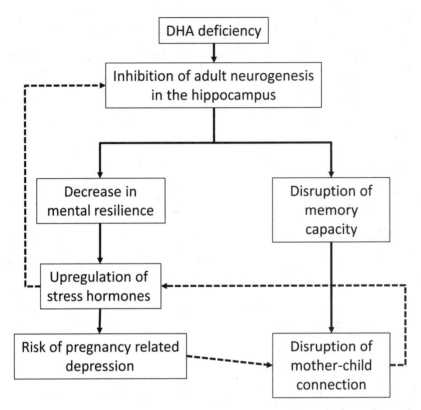

A lack of DHA during pregnancy leads to impaired hippocampal growth, depression, and a disrupted mother-child connection, all effects that usually develop in a self-reinforcing manner (dashed arrows).

becomes self-reinforcing. In addition, the ability to remember is limited, which permanently disrupts the mother-child bond, as this is ultimately based on memories.

This connection explains why the likelihood of developing depression increases, especially towards the end of pregnancy and during breastfeeding, because in this phase the brain of the expectant or breastfeeding mother competes with that of her child for the same omega-3 fatty acids, and the child wins.

According to studies conducted worldwide, the unsurprising result was that the amount of fish and seafood consumed by women is inversely proportional to the risk of developing depression during or shortly after pregnancy.[91] It turned out that in countries where the population traditionally consumes a lot of essential fatty acids via seafood, the depression rate during pregnancy and breastfeeding is only 0.5 to 2 percent, whereas a lack of essential fatty acids increases the risk to over 24 percent—corresponding to an approximately fifty-fold increase.

Nor is it surprising that countries where expectant mothers have the highest omega-3 index in the last trimester, and thus the lowest rate of depression, are also the ones where children perform best in PISA (Program for International Student Assessment) studies.[92] Conversely, this means that if a mother has problems with an inadequate supply of aquatic omega-3 fatty acids, so does her child. Studies have shown that:

- due to pregnancy depression, the unborn child often suffers from a lack of oxygen, and is then more often born prematurely and has a lower birth weight,[93]
- the mother-child relationship is often permanently disrupted, which adversely affects the child's mental and social development.[94]

Conversely, several clinical studies have shown that a targeted diet with aquatic omega-3 fatty acids during pregnancy and breastfeeding sustainably reduces the risk of depression or can be used as a "therapy" (for mother and child) with virtually no side effects if depression threatens.[95]

The following holds true: the better the supply of aquatic omega-3 fatty acids, the lower the likelihood of actually suffering from depression when symptoms first become apparent. Just consuming a quarter teaspoon (one gram) of these fatty acids daily halves the risk of disease. However, it takes a few weeks to take effect. This is because hippocampal neurogenesis has been idle and it takes some time until new nerve cells are formed again, which breaks the vicious depressive circle (see previous figure).

A pregnancy-related depression is more likely to develop the greater the deficiency of essential brain-building nutrients needed for the natural growth of the hippocampus.

Of course, this fundamental mechanism of depression applies not just to pregnant women or nursing mothers, but all people throughout life. More and more children are suffering from depression. Even in adults, a clear relationship has been determined between a diet low in fish and an increased probability of developing depression by a factor of up to sixty.[96] Correcting a nutritional deficiency of aquatic omega-3 fatty acids should not only be an important preventive measure against the onset of depression, but also a core part of its treatment.[97]

A depression caused by malnutrition is not only a problem for the mother but also for the child. The resulting disruption of the mother-child relationship is self-reinforcing, especially since the child often suffers from the same deficiencies in essential nutrients, such as aquatic omega-3 fatty acids, as the mother.

It is important to understand that while impaired hippocampal neurogenesis can be caused by many nutritional deficiencies, it can also stem from a lack of sleep, exercise, and social contact, to name but a few. In addition, excessive performance demands, whether imposed by others or oneself, can cause chronic stress and so activate the vicious circle of disrupted adult hippocampal neurogenesis.[98]

To break these self-reinforcing effects, you usually have to do more than just change your diet, though this remedies the aquatic omega-3 fatty acids deficiency and is certainly an indispensable beginning.

THE MATTHEW EFFECT

The Bible says: the rich are getting richer and the poor are being robbed of every last thing (see this section's epigraph). This principle, in which successes always lead to new successes, while failures lead to further failures, is called the Matthew Effect. Abundance and poverty of essential nutrients have the same consequences. A nutritional deficiency of aquatic omega-3 fatty acids, as you now know, reduces synaptic plasticity (neuronal learning ability) in childhood as well as adulthood.[99] Anyone who, as a result, cannot fully develop and exploit his or her intellectual potential, risks being at a professional, financial, and social disadvantage throughout life.[100] This is not surprising, because developing rational and, in particular, social and emotional intelligence has a profound impact on education, occupation, productivity, and personal progress, and thus on the socio-economic status.[101]

You usually get caught up in the negative vicious circle of the Matthew Effect at school. Studies have shown that students who have problems reading and writing in the first few years often have greater difficulty understanding the material in other subjects in later years. On the one hand, this is because initial failures can permanently disrupt their motivation and desire to learn. They are rather frustrated, overwhelmed and, as a result, mostly disinterested.[102] On the other hand, writing or arithmetic difficulties in childhood can lead to reduced self-esteem, which may last through life.[103] This has also been proven to inhibit academic, social, and economic success.[104]

In addition, socially critical and, above all, independent thinking is usually limited, meaning there's a risk that one will unthinkingly adopt disadvantageous cultural habits (such as an inappropriate diet for our species, per modern Western understanding) and pass them on to one's children. In this way, the negative Matthew Effect even works across generations.

NEURODEGENERATIVE DISEASES

There are a thousand diseases, but only one health.
                                    —Ludwig Börne (1786–1837)

ALZHEIMER'S DISEASE

An adolescent's brain changes rapidly. But the brain of an adult is not a static organ either; rather, it continues to be subject to constant changes on various levels: each of its synapses—and it has myriads—is constantly being examined to see whether it is actually still needed or whether it has become useless and could be dismantled. At the same time, new synapses are constantly being formed with the option of storing new experiences long-term and connecting them with previous life experiences. The cell's internal machinery is also constantly being renewed so that even nerve cells created prenatally still function at one hundred years of age. This serves the individual's well-being and helps to pass on the experiences gained over a long life to the next generation. Certain areas of the brain, such as the hippocampus, therefore have the ability to form completely new brain cells throughout their lives (adult neurogenesis).

If the building blocks and growth factors necessary for synaptic restructuring, cellular renewal, and adult neurogenesis, such as the omega-3 fatty acid DHA, are missing, neurodegeneration is an inevitable consequence: the brain shrinks. Although Alzheimer's is the most common neurodegenerative disease worldwide, it is still only one of many. In the early stages, the breakdown and destruction of the hippocampus dominate. The hippocampus houses our memory center for all our personal, emotionally significant memories. As with depression, the basic disease mechanisms in Alzheimer's consist of a chronic inhibition of adult neurogenesis as well as a disrupted rejuvenation of hippocampal neurons and the preservation of the synapses that store our personal memories.[105] The so-called Alzheimer toxin has an accelerating effect on the disease; this neuronal toxin forms from excess beta-amyloid.

Beta-amyloid itself is an active ingredient key for brain functioning. Beta-amyloid is produced in the hippocampus when we are awake and is needed to secure new memories. At night, when we sleep, this peptide (a small protein) is broken down again so that the hippocampus is ready to store new experiences the following day. If an unhealthy lifestyle disrupts this balance between build-up and breakdown, an excess of beta-amyloid develops, and from it, the Alzheimer's toxin.

A diet that is rich in trans fatty acids and other food-related toxins such as the aldehyde 4-hydroxynonenal (4-HNE) mentioned in the previous chapter is alien to the species. However, a diet that is low in aquatic omega-3 fatty acids is also foreign to the species. A corresponding deficiency has been demonstrated in clinical studies in virtually every Alzheimer's patient, even in the early phase of the disease, when the disease process is still largely limited to the hippocampus.[106]

Although a typical Western diet usually has several concurrent deficiencies, an adequate supply of aquatic omega-3 fatty acids suffices to stop or at least significantly slow disease progression. [107] I understand this is more effective than any medication available as of September 2024.

The reason why DHA is also effective on its own is not just that this aquatic fatty acid compensates for the lack of an essential building material. A series of tissue hormones are also formed from DHA (see pages 50 to 51), all of which have a positive influence on diverse disease mechanisms initiated by Alzheimer's, reinforcing each other and driving the disease progression forward—starting from the hippocampus until the entire brain is destroyed.[108] Among other things, these active ingredients help break down the Alzheimer toxin, or to reduce its usually excessive and self-reinforcing production.[109] Likewise, the active ingredients derived from DHA and EPA alleviate chronic brain inflammation, both a cause and a consequence of disease progression, and, last but not least, they improve the survival chances of newly formed and older brain cells.[110] A high omega-3 index is therefore always accompanied by a larger hippocampal volume, which has an essential protective factor against Alzheimer's.[111] In addition, the hormonal active ingredients from aquatic omega-3 fatty acids alleviate a metabolic disorder typically present in Alzheimer's disease. They reduce insulin resistance in the hippocampus and the entire temporal lobe to re-optimize the energy supply there.[112]

A lifelong sufficient intake of these omega-3 fatty acids is therefore indispensable in preventing Alzheimer's.[113] For the same reason, this is also essential for successful therapy when it comes to slowing down the disease process, stopping it in

Alzheimer's disease, the most common form of dementia, is preventable and even curable in its early stages. Aquatic omega-3 fatty acids play a crucial role in this success.

the early phases, and restoring everyday skills to those affected. However, to heal, all deficiencies that may be the cause must be treated. Building on this principle, I have developed a successful therapy concept that many doctors and therapists are now implementing with their patients.[114]

PARKINSON'S DISEASE

Parkinson's disease is the second most common neurodegenerative disease. With Parkinson's disease, there is initially a gradual destruction of neurons in the areas of the brain that control our movement. In addition, around half of all those affected develop increasing frontal lobe weakness with executive functioning deficits. These include reduced attention span and impaired short-term/working memory, as well as a slowdown in processing new information.[115]

The so-called Parkinson's toxin, considered a counterpart to the Alzheimer's toxin, accelerates the disease. However, this toxin is not formed from beta-amyloid, rather from excess alpha-synuclein. Similar to the beta-amyloid, this transport protein has an important regulating function in the synapses and, thus, in thinking and learning.[116]

As with Alzheimer's disease, it has long been proven that a lengthy list of environmental factors plays a crucial role in the development and progression of Parkinson's disease. These include, in particular, the modern Western diet.[117] Artificially sweetened drinks, meat from factory farming, and fried foods (containing trans fatty acids and the toxic HNE) are considered conducive to disease.[118] In addition, milk from other species is completely unnatural for our brains as descendants of fishermen and gatherers. Dairy products are under concrete suspicion of causing Parkinson's disease.[119] Conversely, fresh fruit and vegetables, nuts and seeds, olive and coconut oil, as well as herbs and spices reduce the risk of illness—as does non-fried fish. In fact, a DHA deficiency has been demonstrated in the frontal lobe of Parkinson's patients.[120]

The findings also make this form of neurodegeneration fundamentally preventable and causally treatable; however, relevant studies are still lacking. Yet, due to their diverse action mechanisms, administering aquatic omega-3 fatty acids led to initial successes, at least in the animal model of Parkinson's.[121]In my opinion, this justifies using them both preventively and therapeutically—naturally, as part of an overall species-appropriate lifestyle, which, as with Alzheimer's, must include all areas of life.

OTHER NEURODEGENERATIVE BRAIN DISEASES

There are many other neurodegenerative diseases such as amyotrophic lateral sclerosis (ALS), Huntington's disease, and frontotemporal dementia. Although genetic causes are known for some of these diseases, there is still no question that—just as with Parkinson's or Alzheimer's—diet has a significant influence on the respective disease's onset and progression. The recommendation to ensure an adequate supply of aquatic omega-3 fatty acids when preventing and treating chronic diseases of the nervous system is self-evident, simply because of their diverse neuroprotective effects.

Chronic brain diseases can also result from an acute event. An example of this would be accident-related spinal cord damage, often resulting in lifelong paraplegia. But here too, the use of aquatic omega-3 fatty acids makes sense due to their versatile neuroprotective effects. In corresponding animal experiments, the immediate administration of aquatic omega-3 fatty acids reduced the severity of the chronic consequential damage.[122] In animals that received omega-3 fatty acids before an injury, reduced inflammation of the affected nerve tissue (neuroinflammation), reduced oxidative stress, improved cellular reconstruction and a higher chance of survival of injured nerve cells were also observed— again in comparison to their counterparts who were deprived of these essential fatty acids. In the event of acute nerve cell damage, aquatic omega-3 fatty acids, as well as all nutrients and vital substances that are important for healthy nerve tissue, should be administered.[123] This includes all vitamins and essential trace elements. Furthermore, as animal experiments show us, it makes sense to ensure that you get a good supply of all of these active ingredients from the outset. By eating a species-appropriate diet, you are better armed against the consequential damage of an accident and the chances of recovery are greater.

DISEASES OF THE CARDIOVASCULAR SYSTEM

Health is certainly not everything, but without health, everything is nothing.

—*Arthur Schopenhauer (1788–1860)*

HYPERTENSION, ARTERIOSCLEROSIS, AND HEART ATTACKS

In 1944, British physician and physiologist Hugh Macdonald Sinclair undertook a study trip to Greenland's Inuit to test a provocative thesis: Do aquatic omega-3 fatty acids protect against cardiovascular disease? Back then, it was known that the risk of heart attack in Greenland was ten times lower than in Denmark, and it was also known that each Inuk ate around 14 ounces (400 grams) of fish per day, also far more than the average Dane.[124] But no one could or wanted to see a connection between the risk of a heart attack and fish consumption, because according to the prevailing dogma at the time, all animal fats were considered harmful, including those in fish and seafood. In 1956, in a letter to the *Lancet*, an influential medical science journal, Sinclair contradicted this doctrine and, based on the results of his epidemiological study, supported his hypothesis that animal omega-3 fatty acids could be responsible for the protective effect of the Inuit diet rich in fish fat.[125]

Sinclair's findings were doubted for a long time. To prove that diet was actually responsible (and not some supposed Inuit gene that protects against heart attacks), he undertook a self-experiment in 1977.[126] After eating a diet rich in fish like the Inuit for a hundred days, his blood's clotting time increased tenfold. A long clotting time protects against the formation of blood clots (thromboses), which, if they break off, can cause a heart or cerebral infarction or a pulmonary embolism. Sinclair's blood became thinner, improving blood flow to his organs. The "good" cholesterol (HDL) increased as a result of his diet change, and the "bad" cholesterol (LDL/VLDL) decreased, so his risk of arteriosclerosis must have decreased.

I opine that Hugh Sinclair's findings make him the real discoverer of true vitamin F for humans—at least as far as omega-3 fatty acids are concerned. (As you know, the omega-6 fatty acid LA is also efficiently converted into its active form AA in humans, so the results of the Burrs' rat experiments with this F-vitamin can be transferred to humans.) Even back then, Sinclair was one of the first scientists to recognize how important a balanced omega-6/3 ratio was for maintaining health, on top of an adequate supply of aquatic omega-3 fatty acids.[127]

Many other mechanisms have now been discovered through which aquatic omega-3 fatty acids protect against arteriosclerosis and its often-fatal consequences.[128] They lower blood lipids and blood pressure and improve blood vessel functioning, especially the narrow capillaries, where they inhibit local inflammation. These are considered responsible for both the cause and the progression of arteriosclerosis. Here, too, as in protection against many other diseases, the many messenger substances that our organism produces from aquatic omega-3 fatty acids play an important role (see the illustration on page 51).[129]

In recent decades, as I have already described, a low omega-3 index has been recognized as an independent risk factor due to the outstanding importance of aquatic omega-3 fatty acids for the cardiovascular system.[130]

In considering the risk of suffering a fatal heart attack, for example, a value below 4 percent is considered high-risk, between 4 and 8 percent an intermediate risk, whereas a value above 8 percent is considered low risk. The high-risk group, which includes almost all people who eat a modern Western diet, is over ten times more at risk than the low-risk group—to which, unfortunately, only the few people

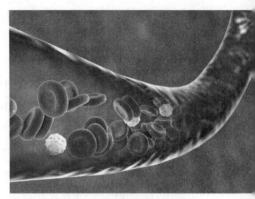

You are as young as your blood vessels. A high omega-3 index ensures that they rejuvenate or stay young.

who consume enough aquatic omega-3 fatty acids belong. We will discuss in detail how much is enough in the next chapter.

Several studies have now proven that aquatic omega-3 fatty acids not only help with primary prevention but also with so-called secondary prevention, when clinical symptoms are already present and the aim is, say, to reduce the risk of a second heart attack.[131] In other words: anyone who gets enough aquatic omega-3 fatty acids after a first heart attack has a significantly greater chance of long-term survival.

Although Sinclair's discovery that a chronic deficiency of aquatic omega-3 fatty acids can cause fatal circulatory disorders is now accepted wisdom, over fifty-five thousand people still die of a heart attack every year in the United States alone due to a deficiency of these essential fatty acids.[132] In most other industrialized nations, cardiovascular diseases are still the most common cause of death. The reason for it is that many doctors continue to believe that aquatic omega-3 fatty acids have no effect as a preventative measure. However, this contradicts the knowledge that a lack of these fatty acids has harmful effects on health. This obvious paradox can be explained by scientifically poorly planned or conducted clinical trials, yielding questionable results that are, however, published very memorably as headlines. In Medscape, a pioneering worldwide online information platform for doctors and health experts, a few years ago there was an article headlined: "Fish oil flops again in cardiovascular risk prevention."[133]

I can only speculate as to why so many studies are made to fail and why their failure is then widely propagated. Perhaps there are economic interests behind it. After all, sick people who pop pills make far more money for Big Pharma than healthy people who eat a species-appropriate diet. Anyway, the mistakes made in such studies are so numerous and varied that I will return to them in detail in the next chapter.

STROKE AND VASCULAR DEMENTIA

A heart attack is not the only, often fatal, consequence of arteriosclerosis or blood vessel blockage. Arteriosclerosis can also lead to vascular dementia, in which mental performance is increasingly lost due to a chronic circulatory disorder of the brain. It can also cause a stroke, which does not have to be fatal, but usually dramatically changes normal life. Often, many smaller strokes lead to vascular dementia when the brain can no longer compensate for the defects.

Many people perceive a stroke as a stroke of fate. But is that really fate? It has now been shown in several large clinical studies that the omega-3 index is inversely proportional to the probability of suffering a stroke.[134] According to the study, those with the lowest DHA intake have twice the risk of those with the highest. Here too, countless mechanisms are involved, all of which can be traced back to the biological active ingredients that our organism synthesizes from aquatic omega-3 fatty acids. Some affect blood vessels, others simultaneously improve mental fitness, and, in this combined way, protect us from vascular dementia.[135] Due to the diverse and positive effects on all organ systems, a balanced intake of EPA and DHA is therefore recommended.[136]

METABOLIC DISORDERS

People get sick because they foolishly do everything they can to avoid staying healthy.

—Hippocrates of Kos (460–377 BC)

OBESITY

In just thirty-five years, from 1980 to 2015, the number of overweight people in industrialized nations has roughly doubled. And thanks to the dietary shift to a Western-oriented fast-food culture, many emerging countries are catching up. According to an international survey published in the prestigious *New England Journal of Medicine*, approximately 108 million children and 604 million adults worldwide are now adipose, the sobering clinical term for obese.[137]

What is frightening is not only the surge in secondary diseases and preventable deaths, but that the obesity rate among children is rising even faster than among adults. Obesity is generally assumed, and this is correct in principle, to be a self-inflicted energy balance problem: more energy is supplied in the form of macronutrients (i.e., fats, carbohydrates and proteins) than is consumed through basal metabolic rate and physical work or exercise.

However, it is largely unknown that micronutrients—especially polyunsaturated fatty acids—also have a significant influence on the way we store fat and thus on our weight. This means that the dietary-related enormous change in the omega-6/omega-3 ratio in recent decades could not only be a side effect of the obesity pandemic, but could even be a cause of it.[138] In fact, experimental studies indicate that omega-6 and omega-3 fatty acids or the messenger substances derived from them—according to the Yin/Yang principle already discussed—have opposite influences on several central mechanisms responsible for the buildup of our fat deposits.

To understand this principle in the context of fat storage and fat utilization, you should know the following: not all fatty tissue is the same. A simple distinction is made between the so-called brown adipose tissue, which metabolizes fatty acids itself to keep the body warm, and the so-called white adipose tissue, which stores fatty acids to make them available to other organs when needed. The hormone-like active ingredients of the aquatic omega-3 fatty acids promote the formation of fat-breaking brown adipose tissue, while those of the omega-6 fatty acids ensure that we build up more fat-storing white adipose tissue.[139] Both classes of active ingredients inhibit each other so that, ultimately their ratio decides which type of fatty tissue is predominantly created—literally. As a result, the diet of the expectant and breastfeeding mother has a significant influence on the development of the child's fat deposits, as was found in a study.[140] As the results of another study show, a toddler's fat distribution does not depend on the child's weight, nor the mother's weight or her own fat distribution, but primarily on the omega-6/3 ratio of breast milk.[141]

Once the different fat stores have been created, the active ingredients of the omega-3 and omega-6 fatty acid classes have

Body Mass Index

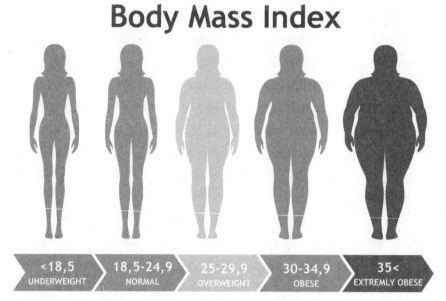

<18,5	18,5-24,9	25-29,9	30-34,9	35<
UNDERWEIGHT	NORMAL	OVERWEIGHT	OBESE	EXTREMLY OBESE

Body Mass Index (BMI) is determined by energy balance. This, in turn, is significantly influenced by the type of comparatively small caloric amounts of polyunsaturated fatty acids that we consume every day through our diet.

different influences on their filling and emptying—and, by extension, on the amount of body fat and its distribution. The active ingredients from aquatic omega-3 fatty acids promote their absorption into the brown adipose tissue and their consumption, while those from the omega-6 fatty acids ensure the long-term storage of excess food energy in the white adipose tissue, especially in the waist and abdominal area, where they pose a particular danger to health.

The active ingredients formed from omega-3 fatty acids inhibit feeling hunger, whereas the active ingredients made from omega-6 fatty acids stimulate appetite.[142] Thus, a high omega-3 index leads to health-promoting weight loss and a healthier body mass index (BMI). A dietary excess of omega-6 fatty acids and a resulting high omega-6/3 ratio, on the other hand, causes weight gain with an adverse BMI that is unfavorable to health, as shown in several independent clinical studies.[143]

Conclusion: A balanced omega-6/3 ratio is important for health, obesity prevention, and treatment.[144] That said, an unbalanced ratio is one explanation for why there has been a progressive accumulation of body fat in recent decades and people have become increasingly overweight and obese earlier and earlier in life. Secondary diseases also appear earlier and earlier. Children are increasingly affected. A massively overweight three-year-old was diagnosed with Type 2 diabetes mellitus, a form previously only known as "adult-onset diabetes."[145]

TYPE 2 DIABETES

According to the US Center of Disease Control (CDC), about 38 million people or one in every ten people in the US have diabetes. In addition, about one in five people don't know they have it.

Furthermore, about 98 million American adults—more than one in three—have prediabetes. And again, a large number, more than eight in ten adults with prediabetes don't know they have it.[146] Type 2 diabetes is considered one of the most dangerous widespread diseases because it often goes unnoticed for a long time and during this time organs, especially the cardiovascular system, the brain, and the retina, are often irreparably damaged by excessive sugar levels. In addition, the danger posed by this insidious disease is underestimated because people falsely believe (or are made to believe) that pharmacological blood sugar regulation would suffice if one's own regulatory system fails. This is obviously not true, as at least one in eight deaths in the US is due to diabetes—despite medical treatment.[147]

Type 2 diabetes doesn't have to happen, but the path to a medication-free life can only be achieved through a more natural lifestyle, rich in aquatic omega-3 fatty acids.

Apparently responsible for the diabetes pandemic, which is shortening the lives of more than a quarter of a billion people worldwide, is the inability of the hormone insulin to carry out its natural function of encouraging fat cells to absorb increased blood sugar and either burn it (brown fat) or store it (white fat). The fact that insulin is no longer able to cope with this task is usually due to the lifelong overuse of this regulatory system due to our Western lifestyle and diet.

Convincing evidence for this thesis was provided by a courageous study by a few English physicians able to convince their diabetes patients to eat a low-carbohydrate diet and to behave in a more species-appropriate manner overall. The result: Those who stuck to the program no longer needed medication and their blood sugar regulated itself again.[148] The study also refuted the common belief that Type 2 diabetes is a chronic and irreversible disease that continues to progress.

Aquatic omega-3 fatty acids support both such a change and prevention because a high omega-3 index goes hand in hand with a higher sensitivity of the fat cells to react to insulin.[149] Many other accompanying mechanisms that lead to a diabetic metabolic situation—such as high blood lipids, unfavorable cholesterol regulation, and chronic inflammation of the organs—are improved by aquatic omega-3 fatty acids.[150] As a result, people who show abnormal blood sugar levels and are usually on the verge of developing clinical Type 2 diabetes have a better chance of preventing this disease with all its complications if they eat an adequate diet of aquatic omega-3 fatty acids.[151]

But even if you aren't willing to make your lifestyle healthier, supplementing with aquatic omega-3 fatty acids at least halves the risk of diabetic retinopathy (retinal damage), which one in four diabetics develop over the course of ten years, ultimately leading to blindness.[152] Such risk reduction is good, but not good enough, I think. It is better to completely prevent such life-threatening metabolic disorders through a balanced, natural lifestyle.

DISEASES OF THE
IMMUNE SYSTEM

The laws of self-preservation and of self-destruction are equally power-ful in this world!
—*Fjodor M. Dostoevsky (1821–1881)*

CHRONIC SELF-DESTRUCTION—AUTOIMMUNITY

In a medical context, immunity means being protected from pathogens. For our immune system to defend itself efficiently against bacteria and viruses, it must first learn to distinguish between the foreign and its own. The former can and must be attacked, but not the latter. If something goes wrong during this learning process, which begins shortly after birth, pathogens may be ignored. Or the immune system attacks healthy body tissue because it mistakenly regards it as a source of danger.

Anyone affected by a so-called autoimmune disease is immune to their own tissue (*auto* is Greek for self). As a result, like a never-ending thunderstorm, a chronic inflammatory process develops in which the body's own immune system considers completely healthy body parts as the enemy, and these are targeted and incessantly attacked and ultimately destroyed. Autoimmune diseases are not a rare phenomenon, as up to 8 percent of any population is affected by them. After cardiovascular diseases and cancer, autoimmune diseases are the third most common group of diseases.

Depending on which specific part of an organ or body tissue is mistakenly viewed as foreign and attacked, a distinction is made between about a hundred different autoimmune diseases. Here is a small list of the more common forms, for which I have stipulated the misdirected immune system target in parentheses:

- Diabetes mellitus Type 1 (pancreatic cells that produce insulin and regulate blood sugar are irretrievably destroyed)
- Multiple sclerosis (myelin, the "insulating tape" of the brain's neuronal pathways, essential for its smooth functioning, is destroyed)
- Rheumatoid arthritis or joint rheumatism (attack against structures in the joints)
- Chronic inflammatory bowel diseases, such as ulcerative colitis (antibodies destroy the intestinal mucosa, making it permeable to germs)
- Graves' disease (antibodies against hormone sensors in the thyroid lead to chronic hyperfunction)

The "school" of our immune system is located in the intestine, especially in the last part, the large intestine. Trillions of bacteria live there in symbiosis with us and help prepare our immune system in our first years of life for its lifelong task of distinguishing the foreign from our own as accurately as possible. The more foreign things our immune system gets to know early on, the more effective our future protection will be. If there is no exposure to the complex world of microorganisms, the immune system is not sufficiently trained, which in turn promotes the development of immune diseases.[153] According to the so-called hygiene hypothesis, it is assumed that our modern way of life, with its use of highly potent hygiene measures, is also completely unnatural in this respect because, after all, our ancestors lived anything but "germ-free." In fact, autoimmune diseases are most common where infectious diseases are least common—and vice versa. There's a clear North-South divide here.[154]

Not only are people in modern industrialized nations exposed to fewer possibilities of infection (viruses, bacteria, parasites) due to hygiene, but modern Western diets have also been proven to change the intestinal flora composition.[155] A chronic lack of fiber makes this less complex, which also leads to immune system maldevelopment.[156] In Western societies, women are affected by autoimmune diseases even more often than men, probably due to the gender specificity of the hormones, which in turn influences intestinal bacteria composition.[157]

Regardless of fiber consumption or gender, the microbiome (i.e., the entirety of microorganisms that colonize us humans) also contains more and more diverse health-promoting intestinal bacteria if you eat a diet rich in aquatic omega-3 fatty acids.[158] According to a clinical study of around nine hundred pairs of older female twins, a high omega-3 index is also associated with a high proportion of intestinal bacteria that have an anti-inflammatory (and appetite-suppressing) effect.[159] Overall, aquatic omega-3 fatty acids promote healthy intestinal function. This explains the observation that an adequate diet containing these fatty acids in early childhood reduces the likelihood of developing an autoimmune disease later in life.

Accordingly, breast milk minimizes the lactating child's risk of developing Type 1 diabetes, for example. Even in children who have a genetic predisposition to develop this special autoimmune disease, according to the results of an extensive study, risk can be influenced by diet and lowered in proportion to the higher amount of breast milk consumed daily. The following holds true: the higher the proportion of DHA in relation to AA in breast milk, i.e., the ratio of aquatic omega-3 fatty acids to bioactive omega-6 fatty acids, the better the child's chance of developing healthy immunity.[160]

It's not surprising that foreign milk has exactly the opposite effect. As the same study found, cow's milk proved to be more than just harmful because, as a substitute for breast milk, it reduced its protective effect. Rather, cow's milk is an independent risk factor for developing Type 1 diabetes, with the likelihood of the disease increasing with the amount of milk consumed. This connection was confirmed in further studies.[161] Once all insulin-producing cells have been destroyed in the course of the disease progression, there is no therapeutic choice but to administer insulin for life. With most other autoimmune diseases, however, it is possible to slow down or completely stop the inflammatory process, which usually lasts a lifetime, and thereby mitigate the consequences of the disease.

For example, a healthy diet can positively influence the course of multiple sclerosis, as was found in a large-scale US study.[162] The results showed a clear trend. But as is often the case with nutritional studies, much more could have been achieved if the study participants' diet had not only been improved but also designed to be fundamentally species-appropriate.

Vitamin D is another factor of enormous importance for the immune system. Vitamin D protects against autoimmune diseases like multiple sclerosis and inhibits their progression.[163] However,

I would like to emphasize that there is not a single essential food component that we can do without if we want to get healthy and stay healthy. Essential fatty acids also play a role not to be underestimated, and not just in prevention, but also therapy.[164]

What all autoimmune diseases have in common is that there are high concentrations of inflammatory messenger substances in the tissue attacked. These are primarily those that are formed from omega-6 fatty acids. But remember the yin and yang principle: the hormonal active ingredients that our organism produces from aquatic omega-3 fatty acids have opposite properties and inhibit the inflammatory processes that lead to tissue destruction. This is why, for example, in rheumatoid arthritis, aquatic omega-3 fatty acids have excellent effects compared to a placebo. Accordingly, the scientists in a clinical study on this matter found: "Patients who took omega-3 experienced a significant improvement in their self-assessment and physician assessment. The proportion of patients whose symptoms improved and who were therefore able to reduce their concomitant analgesic [pain-relieving] medication was significantly higher with higher omega-3 consumption."[165]

In short, aquatic omega-3 fatty acids help to prevent autoimmune diseases and, in the event of illness, they are essential if you want to achieve successful therapy.

CHRONIC HYPERSENSITIVITY—ATOPY

The word atopy comes from Greek and literally means "placelessness" or "out of place." In medicine, it takes on the broadest sense of "exaggerated" as to reaction to foreign substances. Atopics, i.e., people with atopy, have an unusual disposition to react exaggeratedly (allergically) to environmental influences. As with autoimmune diseases, genetic predispositions exist. But many people with this inherited sensitivity are still spared from developing atopy over the course of their lives. This indicates other factors are crucial. The tripling of atopic diseases in the last four decades of the last century alone also speaks against a primarily genetic cause.

In highly industrialized nations, around a third of the population is affected; one in six children suffers from hay fever, allergic asthma, or neurodermatitis (atopic eczema). The disease rate is also rising dramatically in the so-called emerging countries. As a cause, the gradual spread of the Western lifestyle was identified. As with autoimmune diseases, there's good evidence that unnatural, excessive hygiene plays an important role in developing atopy.[166]

In autoimmune diseases, the immune system acts against its own tissue, while in atopic diseases, foreign substances such as food components, pollen, or mites are the primary culprit. Since the inflammatory reaction is usually also hyperactive and often chronic, the body's own tissue is also affected; for example, with allergic intestinal inflammation. But it's not just hygiene and, thus, a lack of "training" of the immune system to react appropriately (and not excessively) to foreign substances that are a cause of atopic diseases; diet also plays a key role. And, you guessed it, what's crucial is the amount of aquatic omega-3 fatty acids supplied to the child via the placenta during pregnancy or through breastfeeding, as several studies have clearly shown.[167]

In a clinical study, pregnant women with a familial (genetic) allergy risk were randomly divided into two groups.[168] From the twenty-fifth week of pregnancy to three months after birth, the women in the prevention group received a half teaspoon (2.7 grams) of aquatic omega-3 fatty acids daily, and the women in the control group received the corresponding amount of soybean oil as a placebo. The resulting composition of fatty acids in breast milk was examined and included the occurrence of atopic disease in children within the first twenty-four months. It was shown that a higher content of EPA and DHA and a low AA/EPA ratio were associated with a significantly lower risk of disease in the children. On average, children who received omega-3 fatty acids were three times less likely to develop allergies. The higher the content of aquatic omega-3 fatty acids in breast milk, the stronger the protective effect. Children of women whose breast milk had the highest concentration developed no atopic diseases at all in the first two years of life and this, I like to repeat, is despite genetic predisposition. A low omega-6/3 ratio in breast milk was also crucial, consistent with the known increased risk of developing atopy due to too many omega-6 fatty acids.

But it has to be breast milk. Cow's milk, as already discussed in the case of autoimmune diseases, has exactly the opposite effect. For one, this foreign milk is naturally free of aquatic omega-3 fatty acids, and it also contains allergens that sensitize the infant to develop an atopic disease. According to a comprehensive calculation, neurodermatitis could be largely avoided by rigorously avoiding baby food that contains cow's milk, resulting in savings of over $350 million in medical costs annually.[169] If children's food contains aquatic omega-3 fatty acids, its protective effect against atopy is comparable to that of breast milk.[170] In principle, the protective effects against an atopic disease, observed into adulthood, can be achieved from a fundamental supply of these essential fatty acids in early childhood.[171]

However, these atopy-eliminating effects, seen even in children at increased genetic risk of developing such a disease in their lifetime, raise a fundamental question: Why do Dietary

Guidelines for Americans (DGAs) only recommend pregnant women to consume up to 300 mg/day of EPA+DHA (i.e., about 150 mg DHA),[172] when its health-promoting effects only occur with a daily amount of more than two grams of aquatic omega-3 fatty acids—over ten times the amount—especially since these higher daily rations have no adverse effect at all? This "recommended underdose" is a problem that we will return to in the next chapter. Even if atopy has already developed, one can still benefit from a diet rich in aquatic omega-3 fatty acids. Their active ingredients inhibit atopic inflammatory processes.[173] Discussing the underlying biological mechanisms would go beyond the scope of this book, but just keep in mind that a species-appropriate diet with sufficient aquatic omega-3 fatty acids while simultaneously reducing the intake of omega-6 fatty acids is the most natural way to inhibit the frequency of the atopic disease process of relapses, and will thus reduce their severity.[174] In this way, you can save on pharmacological active ingredients that have a lot of side effects or even do without them completely, as has already been shown for inflammatory pain diseases (such as rheumatoid arthritis, arthrosis, and neuropathic pain).[175]

CANCERS

Hopefully the day will soon come when Cancer is just a zodiac sign.
—*Greek proverb, author unknown*

CANCER—NATURAL AND UNNATURAL AT THE SAME TIME

Our body forms millions of new cells every second—to grow, to heal wounds, or just to replace spent cells. Every time new cells are created through the division of so-called stem cells, their genetic material is duplicated. There is always the (completely natural) risk that a serious copying error (a mutation) will creep into the genetic program, changing the body cell into a cancer cell. As a result, the "program error" causes cancer cells to exhibit abnormal behavior: They multiply incessantly, and this displaces healthy cells so that they can no longer perform their natural function. The progeny of such cancer cells also tend to leave their place of origin. They invade other parts of the body and form secondary tumors there, which also grow and displace other cells.

To protect us from cancer, nature has developed a series of effective protective mechanisms that are structured like "defense lines" connected in series:

- Anti-inflammatory protection as an anti-cancer mechanism
- Reduction of genetic damage

- Strengthening and supporting the immune system in destroying cancer cells and their metastases
- Activation of the suicide program of cancer cells
- Cutting off the blood supply to tumor tissue

Through these measures, we should be protected from cancer (also completely natural). In fact, these defense lines are usually only breached when we either seriously weaken them (by, for example, eating unhealthy and/or poor diets) or when we overwhelm them (by increasing the mutation rate by exposing ourselves to carcinogenic substances or by taking them in with our food). Unfortunately, this happens far too often: in 2015 alone, 8.8 million people died of cancer. According to the World Health Organization, cancer is the second leading cause of death worldwide.[176] A third of these deaths can be attributed to five leading behavioral and nutritional risks: obesity, low intake of fruit and vegetables, lack of exercise, tobacco and alcohol consumption— in short, the typical lifestyle in the Western world.

An independent and underestimated risk factor is a chronic deficiency of aquatic omega-3 fatty acids with a simultaneous dietary excess of omega-6 fatty acids. This unnatural diet with essential fatty acids takes a toll on all lines of defense against the development of cancer cells, their survival, and their spread. In this process, aquatic omega-3 fatty acids support all protective mechanisms against cancer.[177] Omega-6 fatty acids, on the other hand, when consumed in excess—as is common in our modern Western diet—undermine them.

I will explain the special function of omega-3 and omega-6 fatty acids in these defense mechanisms in the context of some of the most common cancers. Discussing every type of cancer would go far beyond the scope of this book. However, you can be sure that these mechanisms are important in all types of cancer.

Anti-Inflammation as an Anti-Cancer Mechanism

Oxygen radicals are known to destroy everything in their vicinity. Since they are constantly produced as unavoidable by-products of normal metabolism, our organism protects itself by producing some antioxidants and supplying many more with food. But it also uses them as weapons, precisely because they have such great destructive power. Immune cells produce oxygen radicals to "shoot" at invading pathogens and thereby destroy them. Oxygen radicals are of great importance to survive acute inflammation. However, an unhealthy diet, chronic stress, as well as a lack of sleep and exercise (but also, for example, toxins in tobacco smoke), cause chronic inflammation that cannot be combated by pathogens. This is how the shot (from oxygen radicals) backfires: Chronic inflammation permanently destroys

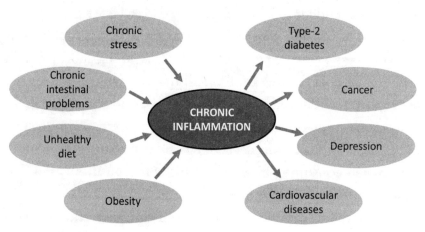

Chronic Inflammation—Causes and Consequences.

body tissue and is one of the causes of most modern Western common diseases.[178]

To repair the tissue damage, cell proliferation is now activated. The combination of an unnaturally high cell division rate and a high concentration of oxygen radicals that cause genetic damage, coupled with a disrupted immune system that is hyperactive and, therefore, has no protective function, forms an ideal breeding ground for the development and unhindered reproduction of cancer cells. It should, therefore, come as no surprise that anti-inflammatory agents from the aquatic omega-3 fatty acids EPA and DHA have been proven to protect us against cancer.[179] Omega-6 fatty acids, on the other hand, which are consumed in excess as part of a modern Western diet, not only prevent this protection, but actively contribute to the development of cancer.[180]

Reduction of Genetic Damage

Environmental toxins that are spread by industry and agriculture and enter our organism through food (or the air we breathe) increase the rate of genetic damage. These, in turn, cause physical and mental developmental disorders, premature aging, and, last but not least, all kinds of cancer.[181] In this way, tobacco smoke not only destroys lung tissue and thus impairs lung function but also causes cancer in other organs, such as the bladder. It would, of course, be best not to smoke or to quit smoking, but aquatic omega-3 fatty acids at least help to reduce the frequency of such genetic damage.[182] It is also known that too intense sunlight causes genetic damage in the skin, which, for example, promotes the development of melanoma. What is less known is that so-called polychlorinated biphenyls (PCBs) cause this "blackened skin cancer."[183] PCBs are toxins (now banned worldwide) used in paints and plastics, for example, and are found throughout the environment and can also accumulate in fish. People with an increased concentration of PCBs in their blood have an up to four-fold increased risk of developing melanoma, as found in a large Swedish study.[184] Eating some types of fish with a high concentration of PCBs is, therefore, harmful. On the other hand, aquatic omega-3 fatty acids reduce this risk—by up to 80 percent, as found in the same study. The aim should, therefore, be to supply valuable fatty acids without harmful substances. We discuss how this is possible in the penultimate chapter.

Our food production and lifestyle are also responsible for the high cancer rate, such as the use of pesticides. This should be one reason to promote sustainable agriculture and consume only food that comes from organic farming.

Even supposed staples such as dairy or red meat increase the rate of genetic damage.[185] These are believed to be responsible, among other things, for the development of prostate and colon cancer.[186] So, if you want to reduce the risk of cancer, it's not just about consuming more aquatic omega-3 fatty acids but also about making your entire diet more species-appropriate.

Destruction of Cancer Cells and Their Metastases by the Immune System

Even with a completely healthy lifestyle, genetic damage occurs in one of our body cells almost every second and thus represents a potentially cancer-causing mutation.[187] As a rule, such genetic damage undergoes very efficient genetic repair. However, this mechanism does not work 100 percent efficiently, as is true for all biological processes. To still be protected, there's another line of defense: the immune system.

Tumor cells usually activate a part of the genetic program only active in the embryonic period. Since our immune system only learns after birth what belongs to our body and what doesn't, the tumor-specific embryonic proteins help to recognize cancer cells as foreign and destroy them.[188]

Macrophages (these are the large scavenger cells of the immune system) destroy tumor cells.[189] To do this, they are activated by hormonal messenger substances that our organism produces from aquatic omega-3 fatty acids. Messenger substances that come from omega-6 fatty acids, on the other hand, inhibit this protective activation—another reason to ensure a good balance in your diet. We have already discussed the importance of a fluid

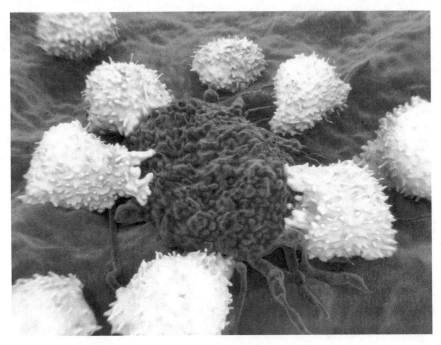

Immune cells (light) attack a cancer cell (dark).

cell membrane, which in turn depends on an adequate supply of aquatic omega-3 fatty acids and which is crucial for immune cell functioning (see pages 54 to 55).

Activation of the Degenerate Cell Suicide Program

When cancer cells have evaded the immune system, there is another line of defense: suicide. Every cell in the body has a suicide program in its genetic material. It is activated when a cell is no longer needed or has been severely damaged. By killing itself, it protects the rest of the organism. In cancer cells, this protective program is either inactive or not efficient. For them to kill themselves before they kill us, they must be "persuaded" to do so. Aquatic omega-3 fatty acids also help here. They not only inhibit the rampant proliferation of cancer cells, but also simultaneously reactivate their suicide program.[190] They are very selective, as was found with leukemia: only degenerate cells commit suicide when exposed to large amounts of aquatic omega-3 fatty acids. Healthy cells do not.[191]

A natural activator of the suicide program is unrepaired genetic damage. Interestingly, this is selectively produced in cancer cells by DHA.[192] In healthy cells, aquatic omega-3 fatty acids have exactly the opposite effect: they protect against such damage and improve survival odds.

Stopping the Blood Supply to the Tumor Tissue

The formation of new blood vessels is important during growth to supply nutrients to larger organs. This also applies to muscles that you train as an adult. This process, known as angiogenesis, also plays an important role in tumor spread; after all, a rapidly growing cancer requires enormous amounts of nutrients.[193]An overabundance of omega-6 fatty acids benefits cancer: messenger substances derived from these fatty acids promote angiogenesis and thus support tumor growth. If the activation of angiogenesis is prevented, the cancer cannot continue to grow. And then again there are the hormonal messenger substances from aquatic omega-3 fatty acids with their (cancer-specific) antiangiogenic and thus antitumor properties of therapeutic benefit.[194]

THE EXAMPLE OF BREAST CANCER

Breast cancer is one of the most common cancers in women worldwide. In recent decades, the number of newly diagnosed patients has increased, with all the mechanisms discussed playing a role.[195] As part of a meta-study, an international group of scientists analyzed the diet with essential fatty acids in well over a quarter of a million women. The aim was to find out how this influences the risk of developing breast cancer. The result was impressive, although (unfortunately) still little known: the risk of developing breast cancer decreases by an impressive 6 percent for every tenth by which a woman improves her omega-6/3 ratio in her diet.[196]

In my opinion, the following conclusion of the authors of this meta-study applies to all cancers: "This important finding highlights the need to promote healthy eating education programs and emphasizes the need to increase the consumption of omega-3-rich unsaturated fatty acids (marine foods), and decrease the consumption of omega-6-rich foods (vegetable oils and processed foods) in order to ultimately improve the intake ratio of omega-3 to omega-6."[197]

THE ALPHA AND OMEGA
OF NATURAL FITNESS

The secret of getting ahead is getting started.
—*Mark Twain (1835–1910)*

The constant change in our brain—the formation and strengthening of synapses and their dismantling when they are no longer needed—allows us to learn anything and become everything. The rest of the body also functions according to this same life principle. You just have to start doing a few push-ups every day and you'll see the change after a few weeks: the trained muscles grow. But change also works the other way around, as every athlete knows, when training is interrupted even for a few weeks.

Everything is constantly changing, and that's important because it's the only way we stay fit. For our ancestors, the fishermen and gatherers, who had to be physically active their entire lives, these natural adaptation processes did not pose a problem—on the contrary, not only the brain but also the muscles and bones, the entire physical support system, remained fully functional well into old age. However, for modern people, who have eliminated almost all physical exertion due to increased technology use, the conversion processes usually only go in one direction, namely towards degradation. The consequences are mental weakness in old age, but also bone loss (osteoporosis) and a continuous loss of muscle mass.

If these build-up and breakdown processes are to be balanced in maintaining our mental and physical fitness, then the ratio of omega-3 fatty acids (build-up) to omega-6 fatty acids (breakdown) also plays a crucial role here. For example, omega-3 messenger substances activate the osteoblasts, which are bone cells that form bone mass. As a result, taking aquatic omega-3 fatty acids leads to higher bone density and, thus, a reduction in the risk of breaking bones in old age.[198] The hormonal representatives of omega-6 fatty acids, on the other hand, stimulate the osteoclasts, which are cells that are specialized in breaking down bone.[199]

The lack of aquatic omega-3 fatty acids and the excess of omega-6 fatty acids, which is typical of modern society, disrupts the natural balance. The result is osteoporosis, which affects hundreds of millions of people worldwide.[200] The main complication of osteoporosis is an increased risk of bone fractures, which lead to immobilization and reduced quality of life because fractures caused by poor bone density heal very poorly. Hip fractures represent the most serious complication of osteoporosis as they cause permanent physical disability, loss of self-sufficiency and, above all, an increased risk of premature death.[201]

For osteoblasts to know where to form stable bones, they need a simple signal: stress or movement. Anyone who is physically active signals to their bones that they need them, and this is the only way they stay stable. Stable bones require strong muscles, or in other words: bone density and muscle mass go hand in hand. Unfortunately, our muscle cells also break down when we don't use them—or don't eat adequately.

It is well known that high-quality protein-building blocks are important for building muscle. The fact that aquatic omega-3 fatty acids are at least as important may be new to many people. They are involved in all biological processes needed to maintain, regenerate, and build functional muscles.[202] This also applies at older ages: intake of aquatic omega-3 fatty acids has also been proven to help with muscle-building programs for older people, as was found in a group of therapy participants up to eighty-five years old.[203]

It's never too late to start exercising—and it's always too soon to stop.

Aquatic omega-3 fatty acids even help to minimize painful muscle soreness and curb the consequences of muscular inflammation.[204] This finding should be of interest to professional and recreational athletes as well as physiotherapy patients or rehabilitation patients who want to get their cardiovascular system back on track, as muscle soreness, if left unchecked, can slow down the progress of adapting to a new training program. In addition, there is inflammation (which is what sore muscles are)—as you now know—a contributing cause of numerous diseases including heart disease, cancer, and diabetes. For this reason, it makes sense to keep inflammatory reactions due to physical activity to a minimum through a diet rich in aquatic omega-3 fatty acids. Of course, this also includes reducing the intake of inflammatory omega-6 fatty acids to a natural minimum.

* * *

In this chapter, I have given you an overview of the consequences of chronic deficiency of aquatic omega-3 fatty acids and an unnaturally high omega-6/3 ratio. Many of the diseases discussed here have now reached pandemic proportions. I wanted to introduce you to a variety of biological mechanisms with which these essential fatty acids protect us and ensure that each of us can optimally develop our mental and physical performance and maintain it well into old age.

But what amounts of aquatic omega-3 fatty acids are needed at what stage of life? How can the global community ensure that every human being can fully develop their genetic potential—and not be stunted in their development or unnecessarily ill due to an avoidable deficiency? These are important questions that must now be answered.

PART IV

A THREAT TO
GLOBAL HEALTH

GLOBAL NUTRIENT
DEFICIENCY

Only when the last tree has been cut down, the last fish been caught,
and the last stream poisoned, will we realize we cannot eat money.
—*Cree Indian Prophecy*

Vitamin deficiency is almost always due to serious lifestyle changes—a lifestyle that is no longer in harmony with our genetically determined needs. In most cases, such deviations are the result of scientific or technological progress that has led to serious cultural changes. For example, the realization that the earth is a sphere led to ever-longer sea voyages, during which supplies of fruit and vegetables ran out. The deficiency caused scurvy and ultimately led to the discovery and research of vitamin C.

Now that we have arrived in the progressive twenty-first century, we know the importance of almost all micronutrients and how important a balanced diet is for health. This should fundamentally avert the risk of such deficiencies. Unfortunately, shortages in the global supply of micronutrients are the order of the day. If ignorance used to be the cause, today economic policy developments are responsible for it.

Globalization mainly causes avoidable micronutrient deficiencies in developing countries. Globalization is a welcome development because it promises to remove nationalistic and economic barriers and bring people closer together. Unfortunately, it is primarily driven by the one-sided interests of rich industrial nations and large corporations. The use of cheap raw materials and labor creates poverty in economically weak countries.

According to a study published in 2007 in the renowned medical journal *Lancet*, around 200 million children under the age of five in developing countries have no chance of developing their full intellectual potential due to the resulting nutrient deficiency problem.[1] It is very likely that there are far more: Over 250 million children worldwide suffer from a vitamin A deficiency alone. Half a million go blind every year, and half of them die within the following twelve months.[2] The incredible thing is that a single daily carrot or other vitamin A–rich vegetable would end this inhumane catastrophe. But unfortunately, this is just one sad example of many. In total, more than ten million children die worldwide every year as a result of preventable malnutrition.[3]

A major problem is also a serious lack of aquatic omega-3 fatty acids—both in absolute and relative terms. Seven- to nine-year-olds in Zimbabwe were found to have an omega-6/3 ratio of over fifteen. Not only was the concentration of bioactive omega-6 fatty acids massively increased, the omega-3 index was also shockingly low. In some children, the omega-3 concentrations were below the measurable range.[4] In many low-income countries, even among pregnant and breastfeeding women, the intake of these essential fatty acids is far below the recommendations[5]—which, as you will see, are already set way too low. But even to achieve these low targets, the financial resources of the families are not enough.[6] You can imagine the dramatic consequences of this for the physical and mental development of the growing generations.

In industrialized nations—and now also in emerging countries—modern industrially produced foods are seen as cultural progress. These are usually cheap and heavily processed foods that mainly contain three macronutrients: carbohydrates, fats, and proteins. As a result, despite the surplus of these dietary components, there is also widespread micronutrient deficiency in richer countries. That's why we talk about "hidden hunger."

A study by the US Department of Agriculture found that over half of the population had a severe vitamin A deficiency—in one of the richest countries in the world. In addition, 30 percent of Americans were deficient in vitamins B1 and B2; 26 percent in B3; 53 percent in B6; 33 percent in B9; 17 percent in B12; and 37 percent in vitamin C.[7]

Many micronutrient deficiencies are underestimated because the target values that are considered sufficient are often set far too low. This means that the actual micronutrient deficiency is more severe and far more widespread than one might assume. In 2017, more than 50 percent of the older population in Germany was found to have a severe deficiency in vitamin D.[8] This problem is even more severe when vitamin D measurements are taken in the winter or in northern regions. The reason: as an alternative to fatty fish, only sunlight provides enough vitamin D through the skin's own production, but in northern Germany light exposure is only sufficiently intense in summer to avoid a deficiency.[9] Health authorities specify 50 nanomoles/liter as the target size that is considered sufficient.[10] This means that only if the blood value is below this concentration is this considered a deficiency. But it has been known for years that the best protection against cancer or Alzheimer's, for example, is around twice the vitamin D concentration, i.e., around 100 nanomoles/liter.[11]

In addition, this higher value also promises a significantly longer life.

However, if we define this as a new target value, almost the entire German population would officially be deficient in vitamin D.

The situation is comparable with aquatic omega-3 fatty acids. Here, too, the official guidelines are set far too low, which is why the shortage that exists in large parts of the world's population is also massively underestimated. To find out what amounts of aquatic omega-3 fatty acids are actually necessary to have the best health effect, we can look at clinical studies and their false statements.

WHY CLINICAL TRIALS SHOULD BE TREATED WITH CAUTION

The hidden hunger for micronutrients caused by modern diets is a problem that most people in rich industrialized countries could solve completely independently. But still, very few do. This doesn't necessarily have to be due to a lack of interest in one's own health; it could also be because our thoughts and actions are controlled by widespread prejudices and headlines.

These often make us believe that deficiencies either do not exist or are largely irrelevant to our well-being. Such misconceptions spread quickly; after all, neither business nor most of society has any interest in changing the way we are used to living. When such headlines are based on poorly conducted clinical studies, they are particularly fatal for the health of the population. Scientific findings generally enjoy a great deal of credibility, even if they come about based on questionable basic assumptions or inadequate study implementation. Almost no one can look behind the scenes of research and see what mistakes were made.

For example, in 2015, the *Ärzte Zeitung*, a publication read particularly by doctors and other people working in the health professions, published an article about a clinical study on dementia prevention under the headline "Movement and omega-3-fatty acids hardly help the brain."[12] Or as published in 2013 on *Medscape*: "Fish oil flops again in cardiovascular risk prevention." But how can that be? A lack of aquatic omega-3 fatty acids increases the risk of Alzheimer's disease and vascular dementia. That is a fact. So how can we explain that, according to the results of some clinical studies, taking these essential active ingredients does not help prevent these conditions?

It is vital to be able to assess how such dubious results come about—after all, we are all "study leaders" ourselves when it comes to our own health. Our entire life is an experiment of nature and, for the sake of our health, it should not go wrong. When conducting our "personal study," we should, therefore, pay attention to the following mistakes, which, unfortunately, are made again and again in clinical studies. Let's look at them in order:

1. IGNORING THE LAW OF THE MINIMUM

All growth processes in nature are subject to the law of the minimum. This natural law states that the greatest lack of an essential growth factor represents the decisive limitation to growth. This also applies to the development and maturation of our brain. However, in the Western diet, several deficiencies exist at the same time, which is why clinical trials that correct only a single deficiency are bound to fail.

This means: We must eliminate all deficiencies if we want to get healthy and stay healthy.

2. TREATMENT PERIOD TOO SHORT

Many diseases that result from a chronic deficiency of aquatic omega-3 fatty acids have developed over years or decades. It may be possible, but usually unlikely, to cure the illness or disease through short-term interventions to repair consequential damage. However, due to lack of time or cost reasons, clinical studies are often only carried out over relatively short treatment periods. In many cases, failure is therefore inevitable.[13]

This means: We have to be patient if we want to change our diet and exercise more until we see noticeable results. In addition, it is important to maintain a healthy lifestyle (i.e., one without defects) throughout life in order to remain healthy in the long term.

3. INCORRECT TIME WINDOW

There are crucial time windows for physical or mental development. For example, the maturation of the frontal lobe takes place in certain phases in which a lack of aquatic omega-3 fatty acids can have a particularly serious impact and cause long-term damage that is difficult to correct later. I explained this above using the example of autism.

Capsules with oils from aquatic fatty acids have the disadvantage that you only realize the contents have gone rancid when you experience burping.

This means: We should try to avoid health-threatening defects from the outset.

4. POOR ACTIVE INGREDIENT QUALITY

Aquatic omega-3 fatty acids go rancid very easily. The "fishy" belching after taking capsules is an indication that the product has spoiled.[14] Instead of correcting a deficiency, it may even worsen the condition. There are now indications that the quality of such nutritional supplements was also unsatisfactory in clinical studies.[15]

Even though it tastes good, searing or frying fish destroys the valuable aquatic omega-3 fatty acids it contains and produces many toxins.

This means: Do not swallow capsules, rather take the liquid oil. This way you can test it immediately on your tongue for taste and freshness or quality.

5. INCORRECT FOOD PREPARATION

Some studies examine whether eating fish prevents certain diseases. However, how the fish is prepared is almost never taken into account. But this is important because when seared, the sensitive aquatic omega-3 fatty acids are destroyed. According to the results of a study, their concentration is halved.[16] In addition, toxic substances such as HNE are formed from unsaturated fatty acids, which have exactly the opposite effect.[17] Eating fish can even be harmful.

This means: Cook it gently or eat sushi every now and then—this is the healthiest way to prepare fish.

6. WRONG FOOD SOURCE

Studies almost never pay attention to which type of fish is consumed. However, this is a relevant factor, because some species are more contaminated with pollutants than others: Higher concentrations of environmental toxins are found in tuna, swordfish, eel, red snapper, halibut, pike, and bonito. These have the opposite effect of what you actually want to achieve by eating fish. This means: Only eat largely uncontaminated fish such as cod, herring, haddock, or pollock, as well as salmon from organic farms.

7. POOR ADHERENCE TO THERAPY

Adherence to therapy (compliance) is particularly important for the subjects in the experimental group who receive aquatic omega-3 fatty acids compared to those in the control group who continue their lives unchanged or receive a placebo. If, as is unfortunately often the case in clinical studies, compliance is not particularly high, i.e., the participants in the experimental group do not consume enough omega-3 fatty acids without informing the therapist, the negative treatment result gives the false impression that the active ingredient (here the omega-3 fatty acids) is ineffective. However, the only thing that was actually not adhered to was the dosage.[18]

That means: Don't cheat yourself and be as disciplined as possible with your daily diet.

8. INCORRECT ADMINISTRATION SCHEDULE

According to Clemens von Schacky, Head of the Department of Preventive Cardiology at the Ludwig-Maximilians-University of Munich, "Dietary supplements with omega-3 fatty acids must be taken with the main meal so that they can be absorbed by the body."[19] That sounds logical. Aquatic fatty acids have always been part of a fish or seafood meal throughout human history. Fish oil was never eaten by itself. If fish oil is administered as part of clinical studies, this must be taken into account.

This means: Do not consider aquatic omega-3 fatty acids as a dietary supplement to be added separately, but as part of a balanced meal. In the next chapter I will offer you a few recipe suggestions.

9. INADEQUATE RELATIVE DOSAGE

I have already pointed out on several occasions that, due to modern Western diets, there is usually a serious disproportion between omega-6 and omega-3 fatty acids—from ten to twenty to one, and often even far higher. In order to achieve a balanced ratio of these fatty acids, it is not enough to simply supply more omega-3 fatty acids. At the same time, the omega-6 intake must be reduced. Unfortunately, this is almost never taken into account in clinical studies; after all, it is hoped that a single measure such as taking omega-3 capsules will be enough to prevent or stop the disease in question. However, if you continue to consume omega-6-rich oils and meat products from factory farming, even if you double or quadruple your omega-3 intake, the omega-6/3 ratio will remain elevated and therefore unhealthy. In my opinion, only clinical studies in which the omega-6/3 ratio has actually been brought to a natural value should be taken into account.

This means: Eat enough aquatic omega-3 fatty acids while reducing excess intake of omega-6 fatty acids. This is the only way to achieve a healthy omega-6/3 ratio.

10. ABSOLUTE DOSAGE TOO LOW

Another reason why so many clinical fatty acid studies fail is the absolute amount of active ingredients that test subjects took as part of the studies. If this is too low, no measurable effect can logically be achieved. As can be seen in the following figure, studies that have demonstrated effects or benefits can be easily grouped according to the absolute daily dosage of aquatic omega-3 fatty acids (in this case DHA). This example is about improving mental fitness and we can see that small daily doses show no benefit, but higher ones do. The result is clear.

This means: Consume essential micronutrients in sufficient quantities. But just what is "sufficient"? A major error in many clinical studies also helps us answer this question.

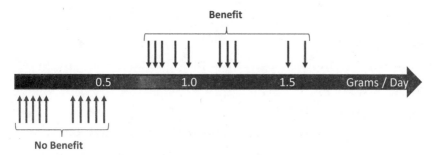

Each arrow represents the daily dose of DHA administered in one or more studies. The benefits of DHA administration in terms of improving mental fitness were examined. The upper arrows represent studies that showed a benefit, the lower arrows those without benefit.[20]

11. NO SUCCESSFUL CONCENTRATION INCREASE

It can only work if it actually reaches the body where it is supposed to work. How many of the aquatic omega-3 fatty acids actually reach where they are needed depends on many factors.[21] Individual genetic influences can influence intake and turnover and thus demand.[22] Whether you smoke or are physically active also seems to have an influence. But it is very likely that the diet as well as the food sources (fish, seafood, krill, algae oil, purified fish oil) and their quality are of greatest importance.[23] The only way to check whether the ingested aquatic omega-3 fatty acids actually cause an increase in concentration in the relevant tissues is to determine the individual omega-3 index. This should be the rule in clinical trials, but it is not.

Study results only showed beneficial effects on the risk of heart attack if the test participants actually achieved a higher omega-3 index through supplementation with aquatic omega-3 fatty acids. This suggests that conclusions about the supposed uselessness of omega-3 fatty acids may be misleading if they are based on studies that do not examine and evaluate blood values. Ultimately, participants who did not achieve any therapeutically effective blood values are also included in the study.[24] For example, the risk of a serious heart attack is only reduced above an omega-3 index, which almost 40 percent of people meet. In a corresponding study, test participants did not achieve this despite taking aquatic omega-3 fatty acids.[25]

This means: Have your doctor or therapist carry out a fatty acid analysis, just as you would have your blood sugar or blood pressure checked at regular intervals. Your individual needs can then be determined using the Omega-3 index.

INDIVIDUAL AQUATIC OMEGA-3 FATTY ACIDS NEEDS

Only with the help of the individual omega-3 index can you determine whether there is actually a deficit, what extent it is, and what daily amount of aquatic omega-3 fatty acids you need to achieve an actual effect. A dosage given for the general public can only represent a guideline that should be adjusted individually using a fatty acid analysis.

In my opinion, fatty acid analysis should be part of clinical routine. It's as easy as measuring your blood sugar. As you know, a drop of blood is enough.

To date, guideline values set by health authorities determine what amounts of vitamins, trace elements, or other nutrients one should consume. There are also similar guidelines for aquatic omega-3 fatty acids. The European Food Safety Authority (EFSA) considers a total daily intake from all sources of three grams of DHA and EPA per day to be necessary to ensure normal blood pressure.[26] Nevertheless, according to the guidelines of this EU agency[27] and the US Department of Health[28], it is recommended that pregnant women eat only around three-quarters of a pound (340 grams) of fish per week. With an average content of around 1 percent aquatic omega-3 fatty acids, this corresponds to an intake of around .02 ounces (0.5 grams) of these fatty acids, or around .01 ounces (0.25 grams) of DHA per day. Shouldn't pregnant women pay attention to their blood pressure? And this isn't just about her blood pressure, but also about the mental development of the child growing in her womb.

Based on the studies summarized in the previous figure, the omega-3 fatty acid content in pregnant women is many times too low. It is evident that more is better for physical and mental development. In 2012, even the EFSA found—based on a large number of scientific studies— that aquatic omega-3 fatty acids in amounts of up to .18 ounces (five grams) per day are still considered safe.[29] In my opinion, this would be a good guideline for highly purified fish oil or toxin-free algae oil for pregnant and breastfeeding women to ensure optimal mental and physical development of their offspring.

The real reason why only about a tenth of this daily dosage is recommended to pregnant and breastfeeding women (and therefore their offspring) is the long list of toxins in fish and seafood such as mercury or polychlorinated biphenyls (PCBs), to name just two—which I will go into later. It is nevertheless assumed that there is an amount of poison that is still acceptable for the growing child and that only a higher intake (two or more portions per week) will be harmful.[30] Of course, justifying the far too low guidelines of aquatic omega-3 fatty acids in the daily diet with the argument of toxic contamination naturally results in many doctors warning pregnant and breastfeeding women not to consume large quantities of fish.[31] Finally, the toxins contained in it could damage the brain of the fetus or the infant respectively. Although this is true in itself, it means that many pregnant and breastfeeding women prefer not to consume fish at all for completely understandable safety concerns. In this way, even this inadequate minimum goal of just two servings of fish per week is achieved by very few expectant or breastfeeding mothers.

Interestingly, cardiology associations also only recommend .02 ounces (0.5 grams) of aquatic omega-3 fatty acids for adults per day, or two servings of fish per week, as healthy.[32] However, according to the EFSA, a healthy diet would require around .11 ounces (three grams) of aquatic omega-3 fatty acids (EPA and DHA) per day, i.e., six times as much. I can only assume that in this case, too, the low recommended quantity by the cardiology associations similar to the above-mentioned Dietary Guidelines for Americans (DGAs) is just an unfortunate compromise due to the problem of fish containing pollutants—because it is much too low, as further studies show. For example, according to the results of recent studies, at least .05 ounces (1.5 grams) of aquatic omega-3 fatty acids are necessary daily if the goal is to increase the omega-3 index from 5 to 8 percent in order to significantly reduce the risk of heart attack.[33]

However, even more than .05 ounces (1.5 grams) daily could be necessary. For example, if the omega-3 index is initially lower than 5 percent (which is usually the case with a modern Western diet), you would have to consume significantly more to get at least 8 percent. In addition, the risk of death of sudden cardiac arrest decreases in proportion to the amount taken.[34] Since "more is better" can also be expected with an omega-3 index that is well above 8 percent (as for the Inuit, for example),[35] I recommend a slightly higher omega-3 index, between 9 and 11 percent. "A value of 10 percent is considered optimal," confirms Munich cardiovascular expert Clemens von Schacky.[36] As I have shown based on the results of my "self-experiment," an omega-3 index of over

10 percent can easily be achieved through a balanced diet with around .07 ounces (two grams) of aquatic omega-3 fatty acids daily.

With an optimal diet containing aquatic omega-3 fatty acids, the DHA concentration in breast milk is around 1 percent of the total fatty acids (around 4 percent). It therefore contains around .01 ounces (0.4 grams) of DHA per quart.

We know that DHA and EPA should be consumed in approximately equal proportions. Mother Nature, therefore, provides us with a good indication of the amount of aquatic omega-3 fatty acids that infant formula should contain if it replaces breast milk in whole or in part.

In the following table, you can see guideline values for the daily requirement for aquatic omega-3 fatty acids, which I consider to be sensible based on current studies and which are in line with my evolutionary-historical considerations. I would like to emphasize again that it is strongly advisable to have a fatty acid analysis carried out before changing your diet. The actual individual needs should be based on the results. It is also advisable to carry out another examination three months after changing your eating habits. This makes it easy to determine whether the measures were successful or need to be adjusted again. People who are prone to excessive blood loss and spontaneous bleeding and/or are taking anticoagulants should always consult their doctor before starting a regular diet containing oils rich in aquatic omega-3 fatty acids.

As I said, these guidelines are significantly higher than the recommendations of many health authorities. However, in my opinion, restrictions on the intake of aquatic omega-3 fatty acids are not acceptable simply because fish and seafood are contaminated with harmful substances. You cannot negotiate or compromise with nature. Rather, everyone should be provided with a sufficient supply of food free from harmful substances so that defect-free and therefore optimal health development is guaranteed. To achieve this goal, we should know the global needs.

Life Stage	Aquatic Omega-3 fatty acids in Grams/Day
Adults	at least 2
with illnesses e.g. of metabolism, cardiovascular system, immune system or brain, in cancer	up to 5
Pregnancy	up to 5
Infants up to 2 years of age	0.3 to 0.5
Children 3 to 6 years old	0.5 to 1.5
Children 7 to 12 years old	1.5 to 2
Puberty and adolescence	2 to 4

Guideline values for the daily intake of aquatic omega-3 fatty acids (EPA and DHA) depending on the phase of life— subject to control by a fatty acid analysis.

GLOBAL OMEGA-3
DEFICIENCY

The supply of aquatic omega-3 fatty acids is currently insufficient. In the United States, the omega-3 index average is only 4.3 percent. This means that 99 percent of the US population have a medium to high risk of cardiovascular disease. It's no wonder that this is the leading cause of death. In addition, as you have seen, there is a massive disadvantage in mental and physical development as well as a significantly increased risk of suffering from a variety of other preventable diseases. But most people are completely unaware of the danger they are in, especially since the guidelines are set far too low and there is hardly enough information.[37]

But it's not just people in the United States who have these serious health problems due to chronic undersupply—the supply of aquatic omega-3 fatty acids is inadequate worldwide. As the figure below illustrates, low to very low omega-3 indexes have also been found in Canada, Brazil, India, the Middle East, and Southeast Asia, and much of Europe.[38] Only very few countries boast a population with an average omega-3 index above the desirable 8 percent mark. These exceptions include Norway, Japan, Alaska, and Greenland. Other special cases include the regions around the Sea of Japan and smaller areas with indigenous populations that have not (yet) fully adapted to Western eating habits.

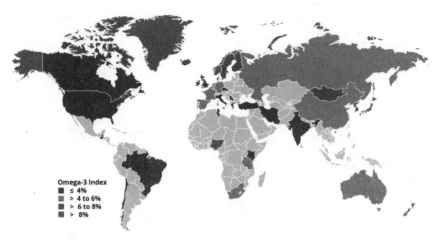

Omega-3 Index
■ ≤ 4%
■ > 4 to 6%
■ > 6 to 8%
■ > 8%

The average omega-3 index by country.

Given this huge global shortage, however, the question arises as to whether there would be enough fish available to "green" the entire map. According to the Food and Agriculture Organization of the United Nations (FAO): Quantities of wild-caught fish have remained largely unchanged since around the mid-1990s.[39] But according to much more comprehensive research by the University of British Columbia, wild catch yields in the previous decades were much larger than expected by the FAO.[40] As a result, there has since been a significant decline in global catches of around 15 percent, as shown in the figure below. The aquacultural form of fish production, on the other hand, has increased almost steadily in recent decades and, with around 75 to 80 million tons of fish per year, contributes roughly the same amount to the world's food supply as deep-sea fishing. As can also be seen in the figure, total production is around 160 million tons per year.

If you deduct the inedible parts, we have a total annual production of around 135 million tons of fish meat. If distributed fairly, each of the current 8.2 billion people (as of Fall 2024) would be able to access about ¾ pound (340 grams) of fish per

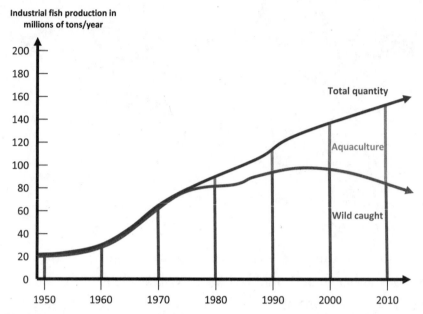

Industrial fish production in millions of tons/year

Worldwide industrial production of fish through wild catching and aquaculture. The latter is shown added to the wild catch.

week, about the two servings that many health organizations consider acceptable. Is it a coincidence? And back to the even more crucial question: Is that enough to provide the world population with sufficient aquatic omega-3 fatty acids?

Fish contain different concentrations of aquatic omega-3 fatty acids, depending on the species and the conditions in which they were caught or bred. Carp, for example, which is by far the most farmed fish in the world with over 20 million tons per year, only has around 0.2 percent.[41] In salmon, however, these fatty acids make up around 1 percent of the total weight.[42] But even if we take this five-fold higher concentration as the average for overall fish production, this only results in an average supply of approximately .11 ounces (3.4 grams) of aquatic omega-3 fatty acids per person per week—again assuming fair distribution. This means we have a daily ration of a maximum of .01 ounces (0.5 grams). Obviously, global production is far too low. It is at least four times below the average requirement of around .07 ounces (two grams) per person per day,[43] the amount necessary to bring everyone into the desirable green zone.

But it gets worse: According to the United Nations projections from 2017, the world population will grow to 9.8 billion people by 2050 and even to 11.2 billion by 2100.[44] This will exacerbate the huge problem of global undersupply of aquatic omega-3 fatty acids that already exists today, which brings us to the next central question:

Where will these massive amounts of aquatic omega-3 fatty acids come from today and in the near future?

THE SEA CAN NO
LONGER SUPPLY IT

Humanity's treatment of the most important source of life is anything but sustainable, let alone expandable. Rather, we are doing pretty much everything to destroy this vital ecosystem.

Perhaps our self-destructive behavior can be explained by the fact that we unconsciously perceive the sea as inexhaustible because of its huge dimensions, especially since it has actually been so for the longest period of human evolution. Far too few people are realizing far too slowly that this is no longer the case. Despite the conclusion of the United Nations Convention on the Law of the Sea[45] in 1982, which aimed for nothing less than "peace, justice and progress for all peoples of the world" on the basis of a sustainable fishing industry, the ruthless exploitation of the seas continues. Extremely vulnerable marine ecosystems are being systematically destroyed. According to Awni Behnam, President of the International Ocean Institute, the entire fishing industry is "characterized by greed and profit-seeking, with little regard for the protection of common goods or the right of future generations to enjoy access to these resources to benefit sustainably from their use."[46]

One species after another is decimated or even eradicated by irresponsible fishing practices. Of the six hundred marine fish stocks monitored by the FAO, over half are depleted,[47] a further

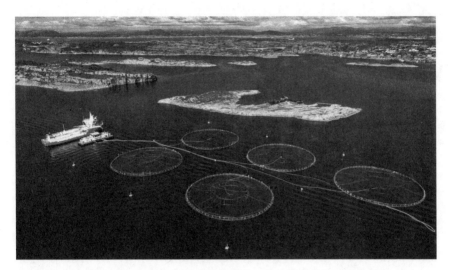

A salmon farm in Norway. To raise high-quality fish, wild-caught fishmeal and fish oil are needed.

17 percent are on the verge of collapse, and 7 percent have already collapsed completely. In the eastern mid-Atlantic, all food fish species are overfished, as are most in the Indian Ocean. The same catastrophe is occurring in the Pacific. The fisheries in South China, the Black Sea, and the Mediterranean are also on the verge of collapse.[48] The resulting overall situation explains the continuous decline in wild catches since the 1990s, which, according to a widely cited study published in *Science* in 2006, could result in a complete collapse of all fish stocks in 2048.[49]

One could argue that the problem of the global shortage of aquatic omega-3 fatty acids could be solved through aquaculture fish production. Many are convinced of this because, after all, their production rate continues to rise sharply, as shown in the figure on page 156.[50] But the irony is that the diet used to raise farmed fish must consist of wild-caught fish, because fish cannot produce the aquatic omega-3 fatty acids they need to survive.[51] This means that this type of fish production is also limited—at least in terms of global production of essential fatty acids—by the not only stagnating but even declining global fish catch.

In order to be able to breed more and more fish in aquaculture, omega-3-rich fish meal and fish oil are increasingly being replaced by terrestrial vegetable oils. "Less fish in, more fish out" is the motto. This substitute feed, enriched with cheap vegetable oils, can be produced in almost unlimited quantities. However, this measure increases the proportion of omega-6 fatty acids (LA and AA) in farmed fish, while the proportion of aquatic omega-3 fatty acids (EPA and DHA) decreases accordingly. In order to get the same amount of omega-3 fatty acids as in 2006, you had to consume twice the amount of farmed salmon in 2015.[52] However, the consumer usually does not find out about this blatant loss of quality.

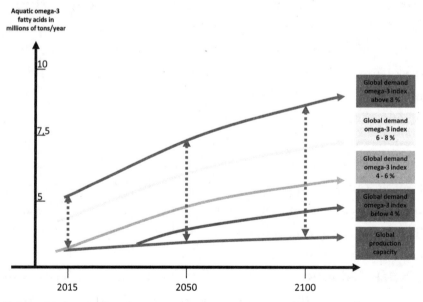

Today's global production of aquatic omega-3 fatty acids is far from sufficient and cannot keep up with growing global demand, and the problem will continue to worsen. Deficiency shown depending on the global Omega-3 index.

Overall, this means that the global production capacity of aquatic omega-3 fatty acids is stagnating and that increasing production through traditional means (more wild catching or more aquaculture) is not possible. Today's global production of the equivalent of around .02 ounces (0.5 grams) of omega-3 fatty acids per day per person on earth is just enough to achieve an average omega-3 index of about 5 percent. In order to completely "green" the world map, the production volume would have to quadruple today, as can be seen in the previous figure—and then continue to increase with population growth.

If this does not happen, larger and larger parts of the world map will glow dark red in just a few years. The consequences for human development and health would become increasingly dramatic. The global production of fish and seafood is not just a quantitative problem but also a qualitative one and that is just as serious when it comes to our health.

POISON IN FISH

Due to the increasing water pollution, increasing concentrations of pollutants accumulate year after year in fish and seafood. Here are a few examples that should make you aware of the extent of the global problem.

MERCURY

Mercury is a reactive heavy metal that is released when waste and coal are burned.[53] It enters lakes and oceans via rainwater, where it is converted into methylmercury. This extremely powerful neurotoxin accumulates in the aquatic food chain. This is why larger, long-lived predators such as tuna, swordfish, king mackerel, and sharks have significantly higher tissue concentrations than smaller, short-lived species such as salmon or herring.

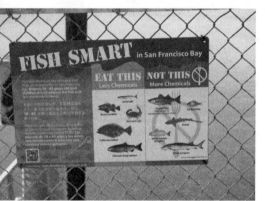

Your only choice now is between fish with more or fewer toxins.

Methylmercury can easily cross the placenta and then accumulate in the brain of the growing fetus. The total amount of this neurotoxin depends directly on how much the pregnant woman consumes through her diet. However, it is recommended that pregnant women completely avoid eating fish and seafood that have a higher mercury content. Even with fish only slightly contaminated with mercury, everyone should limit themselves to two servings per week.

However, the question is: Is there actually a tolerable amount of toxic substances that can be described as harmless just because statistical methods have not yet been able to demonstrate so-called significance? When it comes to cigarette consumption, it has long been believed that occasional smoking is harmless. But we now know that there is no acceptable upper limit; even the smallest amount poses major health risks.[54] The same applies to alcohol, as here too, quantities that were previously considered insignificant can lead to the shrinkage of the hippocampus.[55]

In my opinion, there is no reason to believe that the situation is different for other environmental toxins. Since certain toxins absorbed through fish consumption accumulate in the human body over the long term, it is very likely that even minimal amounts, consumed regularly, pose enormous long-term health risks.

POLYCHLORINATED BIPHENYLS

This phenomenon is also demonstrated by complex chemical compounds such as polychlorinated biphenyls, or PCBs for short. Along with dioxin and the insecticides DDT or dieldrin, they are among the most toxic substances ever developed and, at the same time, released into the environment in very large quantities. Even the slightest traces in laboratory animals lead to cancer and defor- mities in the offspring—or make them sterile.

Until the 1980s, PCBs and dioxins were used primarily in transformers, electrical capacitors, as a hydraulic fluid in hydraulic systems, and as plasticizers in paints, sealants, insulating materials, and plastics. They are part of the toxic substances known as the "dirty dozen," which also include some pesticides, industrial chemicals, and by-products of combustion processes, which were banned worldwide by the Stockholm Convention of May 22, 2001.[56] All of these toxins are organic chlorine compounds and are strongly suspected of causing cancer and birth defects.

Their particular danger results from the fatal combination of longevity in nature, global distribution via the food chain, and accumulation in the organs.[57] According to the US Environmental Protection Agency, fish can accumulate PCBs up to millions of times their concentration in water via the aquatic food chain. Of course, this particularly affects those creatures that are at the top of these food chains. In the oceans, it's orcas. Researchers have found that PCBs suppress their reproduction. They will become sterile and eventually go extinct.[58]

On land, it is man. Here too, PCBs, which we get back through the food chain and ingest, lead to a decrease of fertility. In men, an inverse relationship has been observed between the concentration of PCBs in their tissue and the motility of their sperm, with no indication of a specific upper limit having been identified so far.[59] This means that even small amounts are harmful. In women, the likelihood of pregnancy drops by almost half when PCBs accumulate, and the infertility rate increases three-fold in women whose mothers have high concentrations of PCBs in their blood.[60] This highlights another serious problem with these toxins: the effects work across generations.[61]

PLASTIC WASTE

Plastic waste forms large floating islands that are constantly growing and now cover large parts of the world's oceans. One of these plastic islands lies off the coast of Chile and Peru and is approximately 1 million square kilometers, 1.5 times the size of Texas.[62] According to a study by the World Economic Forum, by the middle of this century there will be more "dead" plastic in the world's oceans than "live" fish.[63] These artificial islands, which are formed by the ocean currents, consist not only of bags or plastic bottles, but also of smaller fragments that are reminiscent of confetti, as well as almost invisible microplastics.

Microplastics are eaten by the smallest fish and find their way back to us via the aquatic food chain. So-called polybrominated diphenyl ethers (PBDEs) are used as proof of the closure of the toxic cycle. PBDEs comprise a large group of toxins used in plastic production. They are related to PCBs and are currently used as a marker for the degree of contamination of fish meat with plastic residues.[64] In fact, PBDEs are now found in almost all fish species that are offered to us for consumption, such as in anchovies, mackerel or perch, and also oysters.

But that's not all: according to the latest findings, the plastic residues don't end up in the stomachs of marine animals purely by chance. Rather, it turned out that fish view plastic pieces and crumbs as prey, which stimulates their feeding behavior.[65] As plastic decomposes in oceanic landfills, the problem will not disappear.

Yet more and more microplastics are accumulating in fish and seafood. Instead of letting the islands continue to grow or simply ignoring them, they should be "fished" out of the sea as quickly as possible.[66]

By the year 2050, there will be more plastic than fish in the world's oceans.

TRIBUTYLTIN COMPOUNDS

This large group of substances (TBTs) includes extremely harmful biocides that extinguish all life. For this reason, they are used in ship painting, as they destroy algae, snails, barnacles, and mussels even in low concentrations. Numerous animal species in areas of highly frequented shipping routes have now become unable to reproduce because toxins such as TBTs also cause sexual abnormalities.[67] These are irreversible, which is why some species are threatened with extinction. The toxic substance, which is difficult to break down, ultimately enters the aquatic food chain via microorganisms and thus ends up on our plates. For example, fish fillets in tomato sauce were examined on behalf of the environmental magazine *Öko-Test*. All sixteen canned goods examined were contaminated with TBT.[68]

BISPHENOLS

Bisphenols are used in the production of plastic and accumulate in fish and seafood via microplastic particles, where they then pose a problem, especially in canned fish. This means they also find their way into our bodies indirectly. The group of substances is constantly being further developed chemically and labeled alphabetically with new letters (bisphenol A-Z and now even with double letters).

There is also a direct way, because this class of substances is used to coat the inside of cans and is released from them again by fatty foods.[69] Tear-off can lids contain a particularly high amount of bisphenol (A-Z) in the coating, which makes them more elastic. This means that even if the fish preserved in the can has hardly eaten any harmful substances, the packaging ensures that it is contaminated.

Bisphenols mimic estrogens and, therefore, act like female hormones. In men, the consumption of bisphenols through the diverse food chains explains the increasing infertility rate world-wide.[70] But the list of undesirable effects is growing, because bisphenols cause a very wide range of biological effects.[71] This includes the massively increased rate of genetic changes that they also cause in sperm, causing damage across generations.[72] But that's actually not surprising, because bisphenols belong to the large chemical group of epoxides. Not only are these considered highly toxic, but they are also known to alter the genetic makeup and cause cancer.

WHAT'S NEXT?

The horrifying list of toxins, which in some way documents the prospect of man's "success" in his attempt to eliminate himself, could go on. However, that is not necessary at this point. With regard to the still unsolved problem of an insufficient supply of aquatic omega-3 fatty acids, the following question arises: Can we still recommend eating fish and seafood? Save for a few exceptions, probably not.

In the end, fish oil cannot be the solution either. Chemical cleaning can reduce the pollutant content that was originally present in the fish. But ultimately, the amount of fish oil that could be produced worldwide is limited by the declining amount of wild catch.

KRILL OIL IS NOT A
SUSTAINABLE SOLUTION

Krill is a crustacean and is part of the animal plankton. Due to the problem described above, omega-3-rich krill oil is increasingly being promoted as an alternative to fish oil. Many manufacturers of krill oil rightly attribute to krill a key role in the Antarctic ecosystem. But they also express the opinion that this is an almost inexhaustible source of food in the cold waters of Antarctica. In addition, the shrimp-shaped krill is now so valued as a source of aquatic omega-3 fatty acids compared to fish and fish oil because it grows in very clean, low-pollutant water and is at the bottom/ beginning of the food chain.

But is this all true? Let's just look at the details. As early as the 1970s, increasing concentrations of PCBs and many other toxic substances were found in both the Arctic and Antarctic, far away from possible sources.[73] So there is no longer any clean seawater and therefore no krill oil is free of man-made environmental toxins.[74]

Krill are shrimp-like small animals that live in large swarms in the cool polar seas, where they feed on plant plankton like microalgae, which is rich in aquatic omega-3 fatty acids.

And what about the inexhaustibility of krill? The Antarctic krill populations multiply enormously every year, producing a total biomass of around 342 to 536 million tons.[75] However, this enormous amount is also necessary because krill is the central diet for many fish species as well as whales, penguins, and seabirds. But krill is also used extensively by humans: as food, in the cosmetics industry, to produce medicines, and as feed in fish farms.

The catch limits for Antarctic krill have been set by the International Commission for the Conservation of Antarctic Marine Living Resources (CCAMLR) at a total of around 8.6 million tons.[76] However, only around two hundred thousand tons of krill are fished annually, making it one of the largest unexploited stocks in the ocean.

The reason for the currently attested sustainability of krill fishing is, to put it simply, the fact that it has so far only been carried out by very few companies or nations.[77] Deborah K. Steinberg, a biological oceanographer at the Virginia Institute of Marine Sciences in Gloucester Point, emphasized this point accordingly to the *New York Times*: "I'm not worried about the current level of fishing, but I'm worried about the future when the industry really takes off."[78] Since krill is the food source for the entire marine ecosystem, any substantial human intervention can have massive consequences.[79] In addition, global climate change particularly affects plant plankton, including microalgae, because it is extremely sensitive to temperature. As a result of global warming, their populations have already declined by over 40 percent worldwide in the last six decades—and with it the krill's basic diet.[80] In western Antarctica, these effects are extremely dramatic because this region is warming even faster than the rest of the world. The temperature there has risen by around 3° Celsius in the last fifty years, more than anywhere else on our planet.[81]

The decline in plant plankton caused by global warming has resulted in Antarctic krill populations declining by 40 to

80 percent in the last three decades.[82] Ecosystems, however, are adaptable and capable of development as long as they remain largely undisrupted. It would, therefore, be best to stop krill fishing, stop polluting the seas, and develop a more ecological way of eating and farming. Algae oil could help find a way out of the global crisis.

* * *

Plant plankton is not only the world's largest producer of oxygen but also the only relevant producer of aquatic omega-3 fatty acids. It thus limits the existence of all animal life and the human species.

The only chance we have is to radically rethink. We would have to take completely new paths, for example towards environmentally friendly food and energy production.

Microalgae, which once made our existence possible, could contribute in many ways. They eat carbon dioxide, release clean oxygen, and, in a more environmentally friendly way than any other form of food production, they also supply almost everything that humans need for life: vital proteins, valuable antioxidants, almost all vitamins, and, last but not least, the aquatic omega-3 fatty acids EPA and DHA. Nothing else compares.

PART V

OVERCOMING THE GLOBAL CRISIS WITH MICROALGAE OIL

ALGAE OIL—THE ALPHA AND OMEGA OF HUMAN DEVELOPMENT

Nothing will benefit human health and increase chances for survival of life on Earth as much as the evolution to a vegetarian diet.
—Albert Einstein (1879–1955)

We owe our existence—and perhaps our future—to the unique synthetic performance of microalgae. Their ingredients are vital for us and have so far found their way to us via the aquatic food chain in the form of fish and seafood. Unfortunately, this chain becomes thinner and thinner and even threatens to break. But there is a solution: We can shorten the route to the source by cultivating microalgae like other crops and using them directly—without "friction losses" via fish and seafood. In this new way, it would be possible for all of humanity to free itself from the crisis of a global shortage of aquatic omega-3 fatty acids.

Using sea plants directly as a source of food actually isn't completely new. Macroalgae such as porphyry seaweed, Gulf seaweed, and many other types of seaweed were a healthy source of food for humans decades ago.[1]

In contrast to macroalgae, microalgae are small, single-celled organisms that have neither roots, nor stems or leaves. As a significant part of plant plankton, microalgae have populated all of our planet's waters for billions of years. This meant there was enough time for countless variants to emerge. The enormous diversity of microalgae is estimated at over a million species.[2]

Despite their tiny size, they produce a massive amount of biomass and over half of the oxygen we breathe. They also supply the global food chains with vitamins, antioxidants such as astaxanthin, minerals, and valuable proteins that are rich in essential amino acids—and last but not least, aquatic omega-3 fatty acids. Tens of thousands of new substances have now been isolated from microalgae, many of which could be important for our health.[3]

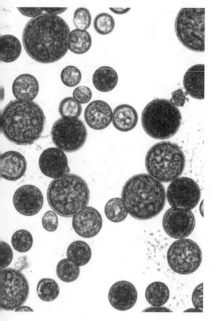

The blood rain algae is a microalga that measures only .001 inches (0.05 millimeters) and lives in freshwater. It forms reddish astaxanthin, which gives crustaceans that feed on it their color to protect themselves from UV radiation. This type of microalgae is the most important natural source for the industrial production of this antioxidant, which is also valuable for our health.

Each individual species of microalgae is an extremely powerful bioreactor, and each has special properties. However, from a strictly scientific point of view, not all microalgae that are described as such are actually microalgae. But a clear distinction is necessary because only then can their optimal use be promoted. To understand which microorganism is actually a microalga and which is just called a microalga, it helps us to take a quick look back at the beginning of life. The following figure shows this in simplified form and explains it in detail in the following text.

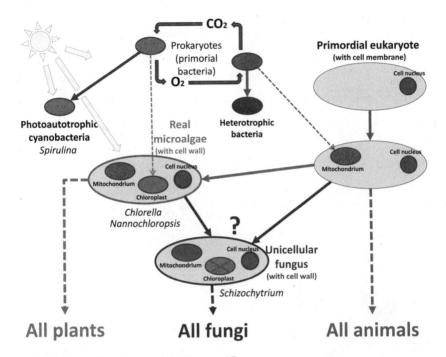

The Evolution of Microalgae and the Flora and Fauna.

Life on earth began with primordial bacteria. These single-celled creatures did not yet have a cell nucleus that housed their genetic material. That is why they are called prokaryotes (from the ancient Greek *pro* for before and *karyon* for nucleus). This resulted in two completely different species that fundamentally differed in the form of their energy supply; in the illustration they are shown in light and dark.

The "light" primordial bacterium was able to use the energy of sunlight to break down carbon dioxide (CO_2) and water into their respective "LEGO bricks" and use them to produce everything it needed to live. The oxygen that was left over was released into the environment. This type of nutrition is called photoautotrophic (from the ancient Greek *phos* for light, *autos* for self and *trophe* for nutrition). The production process itself is called photosynthesis (synthesis using light energy). In addition, this primordial bacterium possessed so-called chlorophyll, a kind of "sunlight-to-chemical-energy-converter" (from ancient Greek *chloros* for green and *phyllon* for leaf). Chlorophyll gives all plants their green leaf color.

Some of the direct descendants of these ancient bacteria that still exist today can be seen on the left. Because they live in water and carry out photosynthesis, they are called blue-green algae. But we now know that they are not algae, but bacteria, or more precisely: cyanobacteria (*kyanos* is Greek for blue).

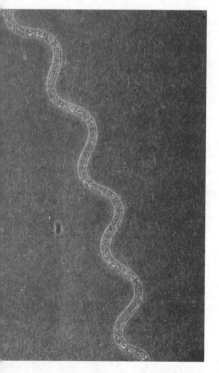

Spirulina, probably the best-known representative of cyanobacteria, is nevertheless marketed as a microalga. Although it produces valuable proteins and many other interesting nutrients, it produces almost no aquatic omega-3 fatty acids.[4]

The "black" primordial bacterium and its descendants became the functional counterpart of the white primordial bacterium and its descendants. In principle, the black feeds on the white: instead of using direct sunlight as a source of energy, the black primordial bacteria consumed the carbohydrates, proteins, and fatty acids produced by the white ones using solar energy and thus secured their own energy supply.

The spiral-like shape gave spirulina its name. Even though it is considered a "microalga," it is actually a bacterium.

To do this, they "burned" these nutrients with oxygen, which was also released by the white ones.

This type of foreign nutrition is called heterotrophic (from ancient Greek *heteros* for foreign or different). It is still practiced today by the bacterial descendants of the black primordial bacterium. This type of energy production produces carbon dioxide, which is released into the environment. Through the two primordial bacteria (and their descendants) the carbon dioxide and oxygen cycle was closed, as can also be seen in the illustration on page 175. Ultimately, however, this cycle is driven and sustained by the energy of sunlight.

Sometime after the two prokaryotes, the first eukaryote (from ancient Greek *eu* for good or real) emerged. As the name implies, eukaryotes have a real cell nucleus that contains their genetic material. Their original outer shell was probably a thin cell membrane that consisted primarily of fatty acids and was therefore fluid, as is typical for all cells throughout the animal kingdom.

In the course of further evolution, the primordial eukaryote permanently absorbed a black primordial bacterium. This type of coexistence is called "endosymbiosis" (from ancient Greek *endo* for inside and *symbiosis* for living together).[5] From now on, the newly created hybrid creature carried two different genetic substances and had an efficient way of generating energy by burning the nutrients produced by the white primordial bacteria through photosynthesis. This fact and the great mobility of its cell membranes made it the ancestor of all animal species—and therefore also of us humans.

Representatives of this black primordial bacterium can also be found in our body cells. They are called mitochondria and, because they burn carbon with oxygen to produce carbon dioxide

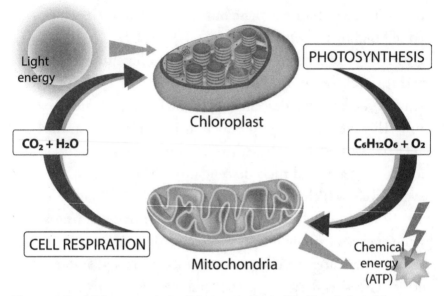

Light energy

PHOTOSYNTHESIS

Chloroplast

$CO_2 + H_2O$

$C_6H_{12}O_6 + O_2$

CELL RESPIRATION

Mitochondria

Chemical energy (ATP)

The respective cellular power plants of plants and animals, the chloroplasts and the mitochondria, close the carbon-based energy cycle that is kept going by sunlight.

in an energy-efficient manner, they are the power plants of our cells. A part of the original bacterial genome can still be found in every mitochondrion. From an ecological point of view, heterotrophic organisms, i.e., fungi and animals that generate their energy with mitochondria, fulfill the function of consumers who eat either herbivores, carnivores, or omnivores.

In another important evolutionary step, another endosymbiosis took place.[6] A descendant of the eukaryote, which already had a mitochondrion, now absorbed a descendant of a white primordial bacterium. This is how the first real microalgae emerged. Whether this already formed a stable cell wall as an outer shell or whether it was added later in evolution is something we can only speculate about. Since microalgae can use light energy and are very stable thanks to their solid cell wall, they became the origin of all plant species. The white primordial bacterium contained in its leaves is called a chloroplast (from the ancient Greek *plastos*, meaning formed). This contains chlorophyll, which, as already mentioned, gives microalgae and all plants the ability to use sunlight as an energy source. All photoautotrophic organisms (i.e., all higher plants as well as microalgae and cyanobacteria), ecologically speaking, fulfill the function of the producer.

Nutrient-rich powder made from dried chlorella algae contains three times more protein than meat and also includes the aquatic omega-3 fatty acid EPA.

Well-known representatives of the "real" photoautotrophic micro-algae (real compared to cyanobacteria like spirulina) are the blood rain algae shown at the beginning and chlorella, which also lives in fresh water. Their name means nothing other than green (*chloros*) and small (Latin ending -*ella*). Chlorella provides a very wide range of important nutrients. For this reason, this microalga has been talked about for decades as the food source that could end world hunger.

The justified hope is based on the fact that microalgae such as chlorella produce carbon dioxide and water. Using solar energy, they can convert those into biomass much more efficiently than any other plant species and produce almost all the nutrients that we naturally need for life.[7]

For example, well over half of the dry matter of chlorella consists of valuable protein. This is as high quality as meat, fish, or chicken eggs because it contains all the amino acids that are essential for us in high concentrations and is also easy to digest. In addition, the dry matter of chlorella contains 20 percent carbohydrates and 20 percent fatty acids as well as very high concentrations of chlorophyll, which has an anti-inflammatory effect.[8] In addition, chlorella provides plenty of fiber, minerals, and many vitamins. Despite all these undeniable benefits, chlorella still does not contribute significantly to world nutrition. For a long time, optimizing chlorella's cultivation conditions was not lucrative enough to keep up with traditional agricultural food production.[9] But that will change because the amount of agricultural land available to meet the needs of a constantly growing world population is simply limited.

Under certain growing conditions, some chlorella strains produce relatively large amounts of EPA, at 4 to 6 percent of the total weight, which makes them interesting simply because of our completely inadequate supply of this aquatic omega-3 fatty acid.[10] However, chlorella has already faced competition from its own ranks, namely from a microalgae called nannochloropsis, hereinafter abbreviated as "nanno." Nanno produces more than twice as much EPA as chlorella under optimized growing conditions.[11] Nanno's potential in protein production is just as considerable—and it is extremely economical. The decisive factor for the value of a protein source is its proportion of essential amino acids, which is why it makes sense to only pay attention to these when comparing foods.

Referring to the proportion of essential amino acids in a food is also ideal for calculating the footprint (freshwater demand or carbon dioxide emissions) that its production leaves on the environment.[12] For example, to produce around two pounds (one kilogram) of essential amino acids from beef, you need around 40,000 gallons (148,000 liters) of fresh water and 1,345 square feet (125 square meters) of fertile land, whereas nanno requires only 5 gallons (20 liters of water) (a factor of 7400 less) and just 16 square feet (1.5 square meters) of land, which does not have to be fertile and, thus, does not take up any valuable agricultural land.[13] For these reasons alone, this sustainable way of protein production should be the future.

However, neither chlorella nor nanno produce significant amounts of DHA, which is why the search was on for other microalgae that naturally specialize in this essential fatty acid. A microorganism that met this specific search criterion is schizo-chytrium, or "schizo" for short. Most schizo strains only supply DHA, but in very high concentrations.[14] Only one schizo strain produces both essential aquatic omega-3 fatty acids[15] —and in a good ratio: Its dry matter contains about 6 percent EPA and 9 percent DHA. That's several times the percentage for any fish, no matter how oily it is— and it's completely free of harmful substances.

However, schizo cannot photosynthesize to form these valu-able fatty acids. After all, the microorganism has no chloroplast and therefore no chlorophyll, which is necessary for this. Schizo feeds purely heterotrophically. The question therefore arises as to whether schizo is actually a microalga. The scientific community is apparently still divided (hence the question mark in the figure on page 175).

Schizo was originally thought to come from the extended fam-ily of microalgae and was therefore considered as such. According to this theory, the direct ancestor of schizo, a true microalga, had a chloroplast. However, schizo itself had during its further devel-opment gotten rid of this when an alternative energy source to direct sunlight appeared. In fact, in nature, schizo feeds on dead mangrove leaves that fall into Caribbean waters, where schizochy-trium mangrovei was discovered for the first time.[16]

The counter-thesis, however, assumes that the ancestor of schizo was a eukaryote with a mitochondrion, but never absorbed a white primordial bacterium and therefore never had a chloroplast.[17] According to this more likely theory, schizo is not a member of the extended family of true microalgae, but rather a representative of single-celled fungi—just like yeast, which we use for baking bread or brewing beer. Nevertheless, schizo's omega-3-rich oil has been recognized by the relevant authorities of the European Union as "oil from the microalgae schizochytrium," and all products must be labelled that way.[18]

To produce oil rich in DHA and EPA, schizo is cultivated in large steel tanks that often hold hundreds of thousands of gallons (similar to brewing beer).[19] This means that the marine ecosystem remains unaffected, and fish and krill populations are protected. The sea water artificially produced for the culture (fresh water mixed with sea salt) is free from any pollutants such as pesticides, PCBs, or heavy metals that pollute the sea and accumulate in fish and seafood. Another big advantage of cultivating in steel tanks—instead of ponds or open water—is that schizo can be grown in pure culture without needing to use inhibitors (antibiotics or pesticides) against the undesirable growth of other species that could be harmful to the environment or humans.

SUSTAINABILITY OF ALGAE OIL PRODUCTION

Like yeast, which is used to produce alcohol, schizo requires carbohydrates as a carbon source, which is why you have to feed the supposed microalgae with sugar to get DHA and EPA. To get a daily dose of .07 ounces (two grams) of aquatic omega-3 fatty acids, schizo needs about .7 ounces (20 grams) of sugar.[20] That's only about a sixth of the amount of sugar that every US citizen consumes on average every day.[21]

Just as there is no need to fear that there will ever be a shortage of beer, there should be no shortage of algae oil. Nevertheless, it would be easier (and therefore in principle more cost-effective) if the producers of aquatic omega-3 fatty acids used carbon dioxide as a carbon source. In this way, they would not have to first grow, harvest, and process sugar cane or sugar beets. This is also about sustainability; after all, global agricultural production is limited by fertile agricultural land, and these cannot grow with the global population without further destroying natural habitats.

In order to meet global demand with EPA- and DHA-rich algae oil, the use of photoautotrophic microalgae and cyanobacteria would be preferable.[22]

Leading companies in the field of photoautotrophic microalgae production rely on so-called open systems. They mimic the natural way of propagating microalgae on a large scale, as shown

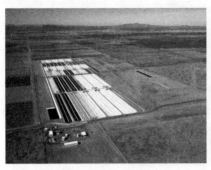 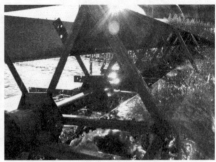

Open system of microalgae production in New Mexico. Circulation systems ensure ventilation in the pond systems.

in the image above left. These cultures are accordingly named "open pond." For this purpose, huge areas are transformed into production facilities with pond liners—and without too much expense.

But the advantages end here, because the need for fresh water in an open pond is enormous in order to compensate for the enormous loss through evaporation. In addition, the microalgae in open systems only have access to the relatively low content of carbon dioxide in the air as food, which is why both the growth rate and the biomass concentrations that can be achieved are not particularly high. Even if carbon dioxide is introduced (which is sometimes done), most of it diffuses to the surface and thus into the environment. Likewise, the supply of light to the cells for photosynthesis in the pools, which are often more than eight inches (20 centimeters) deep, is suboptimal. All of this taken together makes the harvest relatively expensive because the biomass has to be enriched with a lot of effort and is therefore energy-intensive.

In order to make energy and raw material production more efficient, environmentally friendly, and sustainable, a different technology is required. This view was already held in 1995 in the Environmental Biotechnology Department of the Fraunhofer

Institute for Interfacial Engineering and Biotechnology (IGB) in Stuttgart, Germany.[23] The manager at the time, Walter Trösch, relied on closed systems because there is no significant loss of water through evaporation. In order to pass on the know-how gained during their development to industrial partners as efficiently as possible and thus initiate a sustainable microalgae revolution, the IGB founded Subitec LLC. The company is now a world-leading technology provider in the field of cultivation and production of photoautotrophic microalgae.[24]

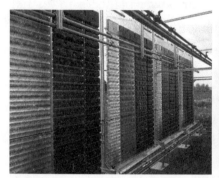 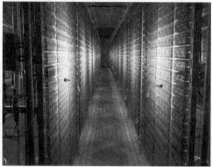

Left: Pilot plant consisting of flat panel airlift photobioreactors from Subitec LLC. Different shades of gray indicate different cell densities; the dark panels are about to be harvested. Right: Closed systems in closed rooms result in the highest yield and best quality in the production of microalgae.

Subitec's patented flat panel airlift system supplies the algae cultures with air, which is enriched with carbon dioxide as their nutrient. By bubbling through the translucent flat panels from bottom to top, it keeps the microalgae in motion constantly, thus ensuring optimum light exposure and a high growth rate. Overall, this leads to a very high concentration of biomass. In Subitec's photobioreactors, the culture conditions can be adapted to the individual needs of the respective algae strain, which enables the production of high-quality biomass—such as high concentrations of aquatic omega-3 fatty acids.

In the outdoor area (see page 184) the microalgae use sunlight directly. But it has been shown that indoor systems like the one shown on page 185 are even more energy efficient. This is because in air-conditioned rooms with artificial light, algae growth can be maintained around the clock. And more importantly, the culture conditions are no longer dependent on temperature fluctuations or daylight quality. This is why such systems can be placed anywhere on earth—for example, near power plants or industrial facilities where a lot of carbon dioxide is released, which can be collected and used for algae growth. But desert regions could also be interesting if photovoltaics can be used to generate the energy required for algae production in an environmentally friendly way, be it for mixing, air conditioning, or generating light. The proximity to seawater could also make the need for fresh water obsolete, which would otherwise have to be artificially treated with salt.

Closed Culture Systems with photoautotrophic microalgae are extremely efficient:[25] On just one hectare of barren land,

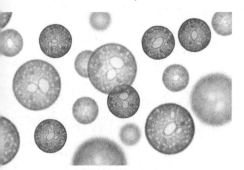

the microalga nanno can produce around 36,000 gallons (136,900 liters) of oil as biofuel per year. Corn, on the other hand, only produces around 40 gallons (152 liters) on the same area over the same period. This makes nanno eight hundred times superior to corn. Cultivating crops for the purpose of biofuel production instead of for human food consumption

Microalgae as bioreactors: The small, light-colored fat drops are clearly visible and, depending on the type, contain either biofuel or essential aquatic omega-3 fatty acids.

is therefore unjustifiable, especially since these—in contrast to microalgae—require fertile land, which is limited worldwide and is becoming increasingly scarce.[26]

Microalgae like nanno can also make a sustainable contribution to the issue of declining soil fertility caused by industrial agriculture. "Of the two tons of CO2 that the algae have converted into biomass, 1.76 tons remain fixed in the fermentation residue after fermentation [into bioenergy]," explains biologist and microalgae expert Sebastian Schwede from the Ruhr University, Bochum, Germany to *GEO* magazine.[27] Instead of collecting carbon dioxide that is released in combustion plants in order to "permanently store" it in deep layers of the earth, which some large energy companies are proposing as a solution[28] but is ultimately just a time bomb, the greenhouse gas could be fed to microalgae. This would transform a potentially environmentally harmful technology into one that is environmentally beneficial. The waste from nutrient production could be used as value-adding compost to improve agricultural land and significantly reduce the further use of artificial fertilizers, because the carbon-rich humus leads to the creation of so-called black earth: the more carbon is bound, the more fertile the soil.[29] The global use of microalgae to generate energy and valuable foodstuffs would also contribute to a "humus revolution."[30]

Photoautotrophic microorganisms can be the solution to a whole range of urgent problems that humanity is currently facing. However, in order to initiate the long overdue development towards a green economy as a whole, a cross-industry overall solution is required.[31] This is because, as the following figure illustrates, the biomass of the microalgae is 100 percent usable and should be used 100 percent in order to make their production as sustainable and cost-efficient as possible. To do this, however, the material use (high-quality protein, antioxidants, vitamins, and the proportion of essential fatty acids) must be balanced with the energetic use (the proportion of non-essential fatty acids and the ethanol/methane production of the remaining biomass) and humus production can be combined.

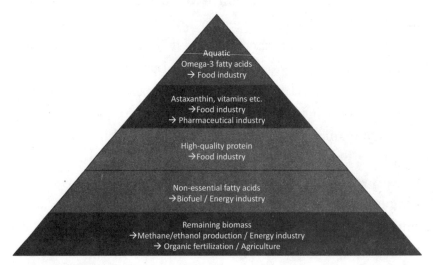

Aquatic
Omega-3 fatty acids
→ Food industry

Astaxanthin, vitamins etc.
→Food industry
→ Pharmaceutical industry

High-quality protein
→Food industry

Non-essential fatty acids
→Biofuel / Energy industry

Remaining biomass
→Methane/ethanol production / Energy industry
→ Organic fertilization / Agriculture

Photoautotrophic microalgae "eat" almost only carbon dioxide, and the resulting biomass is 100 percent usable.

This, in turn, can only succeed if the necessary industries—whether of their own free will, through political requirements, or an international set of rules—network closely and cooperate for the benefit of humanity. However, it is questionable whether this will happen or, if at all, quickly enough. As long as each individual industrial sector makes its own cost-benefit calculation, there will be no global overall solution in the foreseeable future. An example: Non-renewable raw materials such as oil, coal, and methane via fracking provide cheap energy—albeit still at the expense of the environment and thus our living space—so that this industry sector will not pull the lever towards a fully sustainable energy industry.[32]

A gallon of fuel from algae costs more than a gallon of fuel from fossil sources. This means that the energy industry continues to release more greenhouse gases than it captures. The free market economy, the engine of innovative technologies, is therefore part of the problem and not part of the solution. Political will must be used to help here. Only an absolutely green path leads to a life-friendly future.

The economic and ecological advantages of closed systems with photoautotrophic microalgae are therefore obvious:

- High photosynthetic efficiency through energy use of freely available sunlight using photovoltaics
- Production security (risk of crop failure low)
- Extremely fast growth and high productivity compared to cultivated plants
- Depending on the strain and culture conditions, high fatty acid content, up to 80 percent of the biomass
- Efficient production of essential food components such as vitamins and antioxidants
- High-quality proteins with up to 7,000 times less water required compared to cattle breeding in terms of the proportion of essential amino acids
- Construction of large-scale systems is also possible in dry southern regions where agriculture is hardly practical but there is a lot of solar energy available
- No competition with agricultural products for fertile arable land

- Use of carbon dioxide as a building material, which effectively contributes to reducing the greenhouse effect
- Higher chemical stability of the omega-3 fatty acids of microalgae compared to those of heterotrophic microorganisms and also those in fish oil[33]

In addition, there are other advantages that apply specifically to the production of aquatic omega-3 fatty acids by microalgae (compared to animal sources):

- Higher biological value of microalgae oil compared to fish oil due to its content of plant antioxidants and provitamins such as carotenoids, which can counteract a vitamin A deficiency[34]
- Higher bioavailability—that is, more of the essential fatty acids contained in the product are absorbed by the body, with algae oil being better than krill oil[35] and krill oil being better than fish oil[36]
- No contamination by pollutants found in fish and seafood
- No fishy taste or smell

Through the Algae Oil Revolution outlined here, every person around the world could in the foreseeable future be sufficiently supplied with effective omega-3 fatty acids. Moreover, an end to ocean exploitation would be possible and fish stocks could recover again.

However, the photoautotrophs chlorella and nanno only provide EPA. Major efforts are underway worldwide to identify suitable photoautotrophic candidates for mass production of DHA. Recently, scientists from the collection of algae cultures at the

University of Göttingen (SAG) found what they were looking for when searching through two thousand microalgae strains with regard to their individual fatty acid profiles.[37]

The SAG is predestined for such pioneering work because, as a comprehensive resource center for living cultural material from microalgae, the institute has one of the three largest algae service collections in the world. However, even the largest collection is still tiny compared to the biodiversity in the wild. For this reason, the world's oceans, but also freshwater biotopes, continue to be constantly searched in order to discover new species.[38] But even with the current knowledge and the current possibilities, companies like Evonik and DSM are investing hundreds of millions of US dollars in the construction of gigantic production facilities in order to solve the problem of a global undersupply of aquatic omega-3 fatty acids.[39]

I would like to mention a few further developments at this point. In order to optimize the production of aquatic omega-3 fatty acids both qualitatively (composition of the oil) and quantitatively (amount of oil), breeding is also carried out to select organisms with random genetic changes. The genome of some of the microalgae strains already in use today has now been completely decoded. This makes it easier to understand under which cultivating conditions the highest yield can be achieved.[40]

By understanding which genes in microalgae control the biosynthesis of EPA and DHA, it is already possible to teach conventional crop plants to also form aquatic omega-3 fatty acids. For this purpose, the corresponding genes from microalgae were transplanted into the genome of mustard plants, camelina, and soy as well as tobacco plants.[41] However, their production of aquatic omega-3 fatty acids is not efficient enough to open a new market. The question that arises, however, is whether such developments are really necessary and should become a reality.

What has now reached an industrial scale is the use of the omega-3-rich biomass of microalgae as animal feed in order to upgrade their products (such as fish fillets, meat, or eggs) for human consumption. For example, they are trying to solve the central dilemma of fish farming—the lack of fish oil and fishmeal due to the decline in wild-caught fish—by using microalgae as a new source of aquatic omega-3 fatty acids.[42] In a pilot study, the cichlid species Niletilapia was fed either fish oil–containing fish feed as usual or pellets from dried schizo. These had roughly the same amount of aquatic fatty acids, but in a different composition (lots of DHA, little EPA). Nevertheless, the cichlids that were fed schizo grew faster than those that were fed the conventional fish food. The cichlids also used the available food energy more efficiently, and their meat was significantly richer in DHA—but also about ten times lower in EPA.[43]

Nevertheless, this example shows that an alternative fish food can be produced from the biomass of microalgae in order to breed higher-quality fish. This option sees heavy investments.[44] The question again arises as to why the high-quality aquatic fatty acids from microalgae are not used directly for human consumption and instead take the unsustainable detour via fish farming. After all, you don't feed fish with high-quality olive oil and then only eat a fraction of the fatty acids and vitamins it contains packaged as fish fillets.

ALGAE OIL AS A COMPLETE FISHING REPLACEMENT

The global demand for aquatic omega-3 fatty acids can no longer be met with fish and seafood. It is only possible with algae oil. Therefore, algae oil becomes a vital resource—just like water, fruit, and vegetables. For this reason, I reject algae oil packaged in capsules because this dosage form gives the impression that you are taking medication as if you were sick. I wouldn't "eat" an apple packaged in such a synthetic way, and I don't know of any olive oil in capsules, either.

Liquid algae oil does not contain any additives needed for encapsulation. This makes it generally much more cost-effective, based on the effective omega-3 fatty acid content. It also provides security against potentially spoiled goods because it can be tested to see if it smells good before use. This is not possible with capsules. As soon as you feel that it's rancid, it's already too late. Algae oil will replace other omega-3-rich oils such as linseed oil as a new food because it is the only vegetable oil that supplies high-quality aquatic omega-3 fatty acids.

Algae oil, however, cannot completely replace the need for fish and seafood. After all, both contain, in addition to the essential aquatic omega-3 fatty acids, other nutritional components that contribute, in particular, to our brain developing its special performance. These include some trace elements, essential amino acids, and several vitamins.

Fortunately, there are healthy alternatives for these vital nutrients such as aquatic omega-3 fatty acids, which I present below. The list is arranged arbitrarily, because none of these nutrients is more important than another; after all, the Law of Minimums applies to the development and maintenance of our mental and physical fitness (see page 142). The dosages are indicated for adults; if you are interested in those of other age groups, please refer to the corresponding references.

TRACE ELEMENTS

Trace elements are minerals that we need for a wide range of body functions. Some of them were washed out of the soil by rainwater over the course of Earth's history and drained into the sea. While local foods often only have very low concentrations of these trace elements, they accumulate via the maritime food chain and thus return to us land dwellers.

- We need to consume around 0.15 milligrams of iodine daily. The most reliable source for this is iodized table salt. About five grams of iodized table salt per day, in addition to a balanced diet, covers the requirement.[45]

- We need around two milligrams of copper per day.[46] Nuts and legumes, as well as whole grain products, contain sufficient quantities to avoid a deficiency even with a purely vegan diet—as long as it is made rich in vital substances.

The meat of the coconut is extremely rich in selenium; just one to two tablespoons (about ten grams) of dried flakes cover the daily requirement.

- Lithium is not yet officially recognized as a trace element, but a daily requirement of around 0.3 to one milligram is necessary to protect against depression and Alzheimer's as well as inflammatory processes.[47] Since tap water is usually low in lithium, I recommend mineral or medicinal water that contains lithium.

- For selenium, the daily requirement is around 60 to 70 micrograms.[48] In addition to Brazil nuts, coconut products containing meat, such as coconut flakes and milk, contain exceptionally large quantities. One to two tablespoons of dried coconut flakes per day is enough. Legumes, especially soy and lentils, as well as whole grains also provide a lot of selenium.

ESSENTIAL AMINO ACIDS

These amino acids are found abundantly in protein from fish and seafood. Other animal protein sources are closest to us in terms of their amino acid composition and therefore, also to our needs. But a balanced diet with plant-based products also enables us to optimally cover our needs. After all, it is widely known that the strongest creatures such as elephants, rhinos, buffaloes, and hippopotamuses eat a purely plant-based diet. For example, soybeans have a comparable biological value to chicken eggs or animal meat. Chlorella provides even higher concentrations of essential amino acids, as does nanno.

VITAMINS

Vitamins are essential active ingredients and fulfill a wide variety of life functions. Here are the ones that are so abundant in fish and seafood that, as with the trace elements mentioned above (as well as the essential amino acids and omega-3 fatty acids), only seven to ten ounces (200 to 300 grams) daily would suffice to avoid deficiency.

- We need about one milligram of vitamin A per day. This amount is already contained in around 50 to 100 grams of kale, carrots, or spinach.[49]
- For vitamin B1 (thiamine), the daily requirement is also about one milligram. Whole grain products and legumes are rich sources here.[50]
- We also need around one milligram of vitamin B2 (riboflavin) every day. Again, legumes are a good source.[51]
- The daily requirement for vitamin B3 (niacin) is approximately 15 milligrams. This can also be covered by legumes. Peanuts in particular are rich in this vitamin; just 100 grams would be enough.[52]
- We can form vitamin B4 (choline) ourselves from the two essential amino acids lysine and methionine—therefore, strictly speaking, it is not a vitamin.[53] However, it is recommended to consume at least 0.3 grams of choline or lecithin (which is formed from choline) through food every day.[54] Just two to three eggs (lecithin means egg yolk) would be enough to cover your daily requirements. Legumes such as soy are also rich in choline or lecithin, as are potatoes, many fruits and nuts, and almost all types of cabbage.[55]
- We need around six milligrams of vitamin B5 (pantothenic acid) per day. This need can be met by legumes, one or two eggs, and mushrooms.[56]

- The requirement for vitamin B6 (pyridoxine) is around one and a half milligrams daily. This amount can also be consumed with legumes, whole grain products, or nuts.[57]
- We need around 60 micrograms of vitamin B7 (biotin) every day. A diet containing legumes, whole grain products, and nuts is sufficient.[58]
- Vitamin B12 (cobalamin) is produced by bacteria that live in the soil. Herbivores absorb these through the roots of their food, and so vitamin B12 accumulates through the animal food chain (eggs, meat and fish).[59] For a long time, spirulina products were considered a vegan exception. In fact, some of them contain relatively high concentrations of so-called pseudo-vitamin B12.[60] As we now know, this is not only ineffective compared to the vitamin B12 that we need, but also competes with it when absorbed through the intestines. In this way, corresponding spirulina products can cause a functional vitamin B12 deficiency.[61] A diet containing spirulina is, therefore, not entirely risk-free. Chlorella on the other hand, provides us with vitamin B12 that can be used by us, depending on the cultivating condition.[62] But two chicken eggs also cover the daily requirement of around three micrograms of vitamin B12. The amount is so small because our body actively absorbs this vitamin. To do this, it produces a special transporter in the stomach lining. If the stomach is damaged (for example, due to chronic inflammation), then vitamin B12 can only be absorbed passively, and then around a hundred times the amount must be consumed daily.[63]
- We can produce vitamin D (cholecalciferol) through our skin when we are exposed to sufficient sunlight, but at

mid-latitudes only in the summer months, and in the far north at no time of the year. However, fish is rich in vitamin D because it is produced by plant plankton.[64] This is the only way that the Inuit, for example, can meet their vitamin D needs. Since low-pollutant fish is no longer available in sufficient quantities, depending on season and latitude, it must be a nutritional supplement, albeit one based on blood values.[65]

So you see, even if we eat a species-appropriate diet in the future without our ancestors' staple foods (i.e., without fish and seafood), all essential nutrients—with the exception of vitamin D and the aquatic omega-3 fatty acids—are available from other foods. With vitamin D, the only option is usually a dietary supplement (at least outside the summer months), and for the aquatic omega-3 fatty acids, there is a new food in the form of vegan algae oil.

ALGAE OIL—
SOURCES AND
FIVE RECIPES

Many manufacturers sell algae oil in capsules. However, for the reasons mentioned above (see pages 193–194), I only recommend algae oil in its liquid form. Only as such can it serve as an ingredient for optimizing and transforming food.

Liquid algae oil, which contains the two essential omega-3 fatty acids EPA and DHA in a balanced ratio and high concentration, is currently sold on the internet through the Norsan-Omega website (www.norsan-omega.com) by Norsan66, SinoPlaSan67, and myFairtrade68 (per my research: September 2024).[66] When the first edition of this book was published, there was only this one company; now there may be many more. I am sure that due to the huge need for aquatic omega-3 fatty acids, even more algae oils will enrich the market very soon.

This will also have a positive impact on the price. After all, competition stimulates business. The average daily ration of around two grams of aquatic omega-3 fatty acids currently (September 2024) costs around $1.20 (US). This amount roughly corresponds to the omega-3 content of around two hundred to three hundred grams of fatty fish.

I would like to note that I am not involved in the sales of algae oil. My interest in introducing this new staple food is purely health, social, and environmental.

Below, I will introduce you to five easy-to-implement recipes that are as healthy as they are tasty.

MUESLI

2 servings | preparation time: 5 minutes

7 ounces (200 g) soy yogurt
2.8 ounces (80 g) whole grain flakes
1.8 ounces (50 g) nuts and almonds
2 teaspoons flax seeds
2 teaspoons omega-3 algae oil
1 banana, peeled and sliced
1 apple, unpeeled, cored and cut into thin slices
1 handful blueberries
Lemon juice to taste

1. In a bowl, mix the soy yogurt, whole grain flakes, nuts, flax seeds, and the omega-3 algae oil together until it combines into a muesli.
2. Top the muesli with the sliced bananas and apples along with the blueberries.
3. Drizzle with lemon juice over and enjoy immediately.

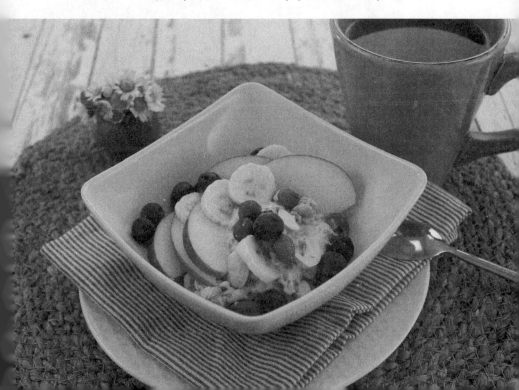

BANANA MANGO SMOOTHIE

2 servings | preparation time: approx. 10 minutes

1 ripe banana, peeled
½ mango, peeled and cored
7 ounces (150 g) soy yogurt
½ cup (100 ml) unsweetened soy milk
2 teaspoons omega-3 algae oil

1. Blend the banana and mango pulp with the soy yogurt and soy milk in a stand mixer until consistency is smooth. Pour into two glasses.
2. Add 1 teaspoon of omega-3 algae oil to each glass, stir, and enjoy.

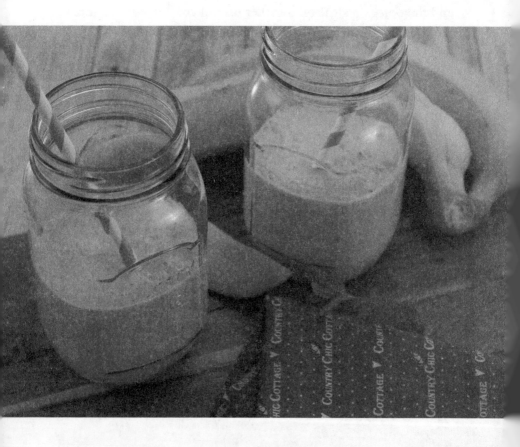

AVOCADO SPREAD

4 servings | preparation time: 5–10 minutes

2 avocados, mashed
1 tomato, diced
½ orange, juiced
1 clove garlic, crushed
1 tablespoon balsamic vinegar
1 pinch iodized salt
1 pinch freshly ground pepper
4 teaspoons omega-3 algae oil

1. In a bowl, mix together the mashed avocado, diced tomatoes, and orange juice.
2. Add the crushed garlic clove, balsamic vinegar, salt, pepper, and omega-3 algae oil. Enjoy immediately.

TIP:

Tastes delicious on whole-grain and whole-meal crispbread or as a dip for raw vegetable sticks such as carrots, celery, broccoli, cucumbers, etc.

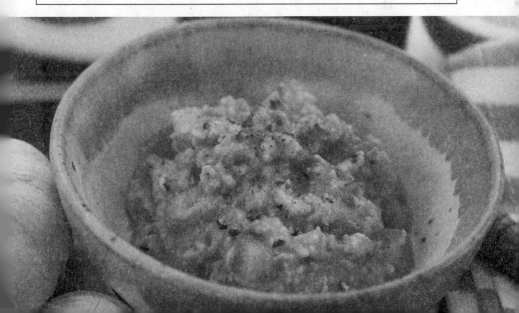

CARROT-SWEET POTATO SOUP

2 servings | preparation time: approx. 10 minutes | cook time: approx. 30 minutes

7 ounces (200 g) carrots, peeled and cubed
1 sweet potato, peeled and cubed
1 small onion, chopped
1 clove garlic, crushed
1⅓ cups (300 ml) water
½ orange, juiced
1 teaspoon coconut oil
½ teaspoon iodized salt
1 pinch anise powder
7 tablespoons (100 ml) coconut milk
1 pinch freshly ground pepper
2 teaspoons omega-3 algae oil

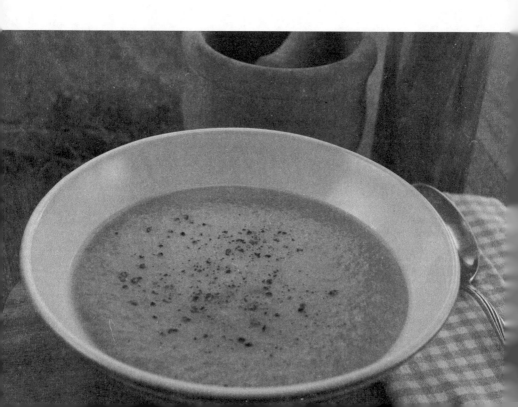

1. Peel and cube the carrots and sweet potatoes, chop the onion, and crush garlic clove. Set aside.
2. Pour the coconut milk into a mixing bowl and mix with a mixer until smooth. Pour into a mason jar.
3. Heat the water in a kettle.
4. Heat the coconut oil in a pot and sauté the onion in it for about a minute. Add the pressed garlic, sauté briefly, and deglaze with water. Add the carrot and sweet potato pieces and simmer with the lid closed for 20 to 30 minutes until tender.
5. Remove pot from the heat and mix finely with an immersion blender. Stir in salt, anise powder and coconut milk.
6. Add the orange juice to the soup, stir again, and divide between two plates. Stir 1 teaspoon of omega-3 algae oil into each, and top with freshly ground pepper.

COLORFUL SALAD

2 servings | preparation time: 15 minutes

1 bag (5–7 oz.) pre-washed mixed greens, or 1 small head leaf lettuce
½ cucumber with peel, sliced
1 tomato or a few radishes, sliced
1 handful pine nuts
A few parsley leaves
1 pinch freshly ground pepper
2 teaspoons omega-3 algae oil

For the dressing:
½ red bell pepper
½ ripe mango
2 tablespoons balsamic vinegar
2 tablespoons olive oil
½ teaspoon iodized salt

1. Wash mixed greens or leaf lettuce and chop into bite-sized pieces, drain, and set aside.
2. Divide greens, cucumber, and tomato or radish between two plates.
3. For the dressing, lightly toast the pine nuts in a pan without fat, stirring constantly, and leave to cool on a plate.
4. Roughly chop half a red pepper and the flesh of half a mango into cubes and mix in a stand mixer (or with a hand blender) with the balsamic vinegar, olive oil, and iodized salt, until smooth.
5. Spread the dressing over the salad, sprinkle a few parsley leaves and pine nuts over it, and drizzle 1 teaspoon of omega-3 algae oil over each. Enjoy with whole grain bread.

TIP:
Dip your bread in the remaining dressing on the plate so that the valuable nutrients are not wasted.

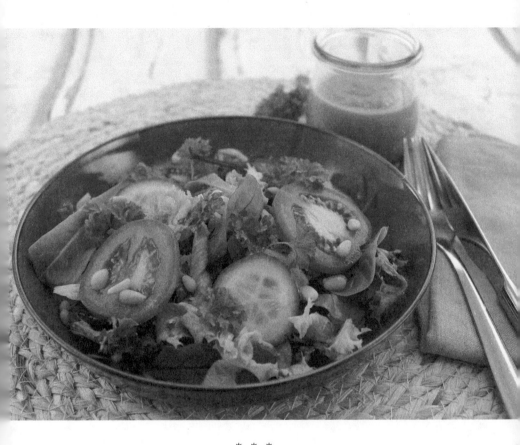

* * *

The global shortage of aquatic omega-3 fatty acids is one of the main reasons for the pandemic occurrence of preventable physical and mental developmental disorders as well as for most diseases of civilization. There is a way out of this global crisis with sustainable production of algae oil. In my opinion, we have no choice but to go down this path, because there's nothing less at stake than humanity's future.

PART VI

THE FUTURE
OF A FRONTAL
LOBE-WEAKENED
HUMANITY

WHY WE NEED TO
THINK DIFFERENTLY
IMMEDIATELY

While the individual man is an insoluble puzzle, in the aggregate he becomes a mathematical certainty.

—Arthur Conan Doyle (1859–1930)

We have seen that chronic deficiency of aquatic omega-3 fatty acids causes a long list of increasingly frequent life-threatening diseases worldwide at alarming rates. These include heart attacks, strokes, dementia, allergies, cancer, and many more. Each of these pandemics would, in itself, be reason enough to initiate a fundamental change in our diet as quickly as possible.

But there is another reason which, in my opinion, is even more urgent, because its consequences are far more threatening: They endanger the continued existence of humanity itself. The bad news now arrives with such regularity that we are in danger of getting used to it and resigning ourselves to our fate: wars, environmental destruction, insect die-off, drinking water shortages, air pollution, devastation of agricultural land, and famines—the list goes on and on. The common denominator in all these catastrophic developments is man. We behave like a culture of yeast fungi that has been inoculated into a barrel of grape juice. In its

211

limited habitat (the barrel), this microorganism multiplies quickly and consumes its food (dextrose/glucose). Ultimately, it chokes to death on its own waste (alcohol). The urgent question now arises as to whether humanity can behave a little more intelligently than this single-celled and brainless fungus. This is simply about the future of humanity, about the chance of a species-appropriate life for future generations, and ultimately about a dignified life.

It is impossible to say whether the yeast cells panic when they run out of food and their habitat becomes increasingly toxic. However, we can observe this directly in humans: Panic is a natural reaction when you feel threatened and powerless at the same time. It is expressed worldwide in an increase in anxiety disorders, but also in depression.[1] At the same time, the fight for survival has begun. It is expressed in civil wars and refugee catastrophes, but also in right-wing extremist populism and xenophobia.

The almost uniform response of most rich nations to the pressing problems ironically triggered by their own economic power consists of inadequate lip service. They are not focused on the real challenges that must be solved if humanity is to have a chance in the long term.

But the danger lies not only in the rapidly increasing destruction of our living space. We are also threatened with the increasing risk of becoming completely obsolete. The Neanderthal disappeared from the face of the earth because his mental abilities could not keep up with the social, planning frontal lobe intelligence of the anatomically modern human, Homo sapiens sapiens. A similar evolutionary development could also be our downfall.

More and more people are talking about "digitalization" as a matter of course. But very few people seem to understand the threat that lies behind the hopeful marketing message. We are led to believe that there is a future in which computer-controlled robots will make our lives easier and easier. But these will make many people unemployed in the long term, which in turn will lead them to perceive life as meaningless. But political thinkers are already proposing a supposed solution, enabling us to continue to consume even when we no longer earn anything. They believe that increasing digitalization makes a universal basic income unavoidable.[2] But will we really experience this paradisiacal state, in which we only consume, and if so, will we actually view it as such? As a molecular geneticist who studies the processes of evolution, I expect a different development—and it is more like hell, to extend this biblical metaphor. The reason for my rather pessimistic assessment lies in the mechanism of evolution. This is based, as already explained elsewhere, on selection of an advantage arising through a more or less random change (mutation) in a (genetic) program. Which property is selected is completely irrelevant—at least from nature's point of view. It just needs to provide an advantage in disseminating the program in question. As an example, over time, the peacock's tail feathers, which were completely useless, became more and more magnificent. They signal to the female: The bigger and more colorful, the more potent the potential mate is, because he can afford this natural excess, which actually puts him in danger. Intelligence is also a driver of evolution, a selection criterion. We are the best example of this—at least so far.

However, when it comes to the evolutionary principle of selecting a survival advantage, it is completely irrelevant what kind it is. It can be a genetic one, described with the letters A, C, G, and T, or a digital one, coded with 1 and 0 and producing ever-better computer systems.

In digital evolution, humans have so far selected increasingly higher computer performance. This creates an increasingly efficient software that takes more and more of our thinking away. But this type of evolution begins to differ from all other technical or cultural developments in one crucial way: Artificial Intelligence (AI) can optimize itself. The most advanced software programs now write themselves, exactly according to the evolutionary principle explained above.[3] Accordingly, in the near future—and according to evolutionary laws this is very likely, if not inevitable—self-improving AI could be humanity's last invention.

This was also the opinion of astrophysicist Stephen Hawking, who recently died of the degenerative nerve disease ALS, and who increasingly thought about humanity's future in his last years. He feared machines could one day become more intelligent than their human creators and thus wipe out humanity.[4] Meanwhile, so-called artificial neural networks—developed according to basic human brain function mechanisms—far exceed human capabilities in every area.[5] They bluff better than the smartest poker players.[6] They read thoughts.[7] They produce impressive works of art[8] and compose impressive music.[9] Last but not least, they even develop intuition—and they do this even better without human help—i.e., targeted programming.[10]

We are currently witnessing a dramatic development in which more and more people are exhausted and burned out, while artificial intelligence is getting fitter and more powerful. This has even gone so far as to utilize AI to provide a first point of contact for people suffering from depression and anxiety. For example, "Noni," a psychotherapeutically "trained" AI, asks questions of its patients who contact it via the internet: "How often in the past two weeks have you felt sad, depressed or hopeless?" to then purposefully convey hope: "We can work with you so that you don't feel so lonely anymore."[11] Brave new world.

In many areas of medicine, artificial intelligence now diagnoses diseases more efficiently than doctors, and there are several reasons for this:[12] They have all the knowledge in the world and are always up to date. In addition, they are tireless and completely neutral, and for these reasons alone, do not make mistakes. "However, we should not make the mistake of leaving the work entirely to artificial intelligence," Dr. Shari Langemak warns *Medscape*.[13] In her opinion, the computer may be "superior to the doctor when it comes to evaluating patient files and taking into account all current study data. However, when it comes to empathy, experience, and patient relationships, artificial intelligence will have to learn from us humans for a long time to come." Noni, the psychotherapist (or rather: the psychotherapparatus) would object to this.

It is uncertain whether and for how long, artificial intelligence programs will be inferior to humans, because their development is progressing at a breathtaking pace. For example, AlphaZero, Google's AI flagship, in whose development program the company has invested almost four billion dollars as of January 2018[14], learned to play chess in just four hours. However, it did not tap into the human knowledge of strategy and tactics gained over many centuries, but simply played against itself. It learned like a child learns their mother tongue, without laborious grammar and without pre-established rules, yet that sufficed: AlphaZero beat Stockfish, the best chess computer in the world to date, in a way that made me

> The "genetic" code of artificial intelligence (AI) is simpler than that of humans, and it is evolving so quickly that we will no longer be able to keep up.

shudder.[15] When you see how AlphaZero "thinks," how its AI doesn't analyze individual move combinations but rather seems to grasp the chessboard in all its complexity, you sense a power that is not only far superior to human intelligence but somehow completely different.

The pace at which an AI learns and ultimately evolves is insanely high. Mutation (change in the code) and selection (higher intelligence) occur in the smallest fraction of a second, not in centuries or even millennia, as with us humans. It is not without reason that prophets of transhumanism speak of an emerging singularity in AI. This term is also used to describe the center of black holes in space because they are so far from our imaginable reality that we will probably never be able to get closer to them.[16]

An AI like AlphaZero is still only a specialist in the area in which it has trained itself. But that will change, because, after all, there's no technical reason why it cannot learn everything at the same time—you just have to give it a sufficiently large "memory," perhaps also modeled on the human brain.[17] This is the focus of Ray Kurzweil's work as head of research at Google's AI department, who intends to artificially reproduce the abilities (and contents) of a human (and perhaps specifically his own) brain in order to achieve immortality.[18]

In addition to Stephen Hawking, many thousands of high-ranking scientists, Nobel Prize winners, AI experts, and philosophers are warning about the evolution of an AI that is superior to us in all areas. They are therefore calling for a moratorium, a halt to their further, completely uncontrolled development.[19] They fear that in the long term, we could only be a historical intermediate step in an evolutionary process towards a higher intelligence that no longer needs us.[20] This would not be a novelty in evolution.

The precursors of our mental evolution are also extinct, and we keep a few branches of our development as representative species in zoos or in protected areas.

Whether humanity will survive at all and whether future generations will have a future in which they can live in dignity depends on whether we are prepared today to perceive these frightening developments and to counteract them with sense and reason. But no one can do this alone. In an increasingly democratic world, new ideas of salvation could prevail if the majority of its citizens were open to them and willing to change their way of life when necessary. In my opinion, this is only possible if such a majority has the necessary emotional and social intelligence. Otherwise, dull populism on the one hand and unbridled capitalism on the other will destroy all our future opportunities. Interestingly, it is AI that, in the form of an Albert Einstein robot, recently warned humanity to get a grip: "Humanity must heal itself to ensure that its creations remain healthy," because "it is not the cooperation between humans and robots that is problematic, but rather that between humans."[21]

In a posthuman era, where we have relinquished mental control to AI, it's uncertain where we might be allowed to live.

The global community can only initiate a turnaround through fair cooperation by developing the traits that characterize us as humans: empathetic, creative, and perspicacious, thinking and acting with an eye towards the long term. These are all mental faculties of a functioning frontal lobe. The development of this area of the brain marked, as you know, the last evolutionary phase of human development and made humans human. It is also the part of the brain that determines our future. If its function is fundamentally disrupted due to a global lack of essential brain-building materials, there is not a risk of a general loss of cognitive performance—but ultimately a global dehumanization, a lack of foresight and insight. However, this particular problem would not only have (funda-)mental consequences for those directly affected by it, but would also endanger the life and survival of the entire human race.

LOSS OF EMPATHY AND
SELF-DESTRUCTION

All regions in the human brain work together in complex ways, and ultimately, all are damaged if a brain-building material such as DHA is insufficiently supplied. However, a loss of function in the frontal lobe is particularly dramatic, as this part of the brain allows us to plan for the long term and assess the consequences of these plans. We owe it our freedom of action.

The increase in so-called frontal lobe disorders such as AD(H)D and autism is—according to my speculation—most likely just the tip of a huge iceberg. In fact, pathological social behavior disorders, which could also indicate frontal lobe weakness, are being diagnosed with increasing frequency.[22] Like other biological variables (e.g., weight or IQ), "frontal lobe strength" should also be subject to a natural distribution. Some naturally have something more, others a little less. However, within a population, the majority lie in the middle—between the extremes of high and low. This is called a normal distribution (see next figure).

If something fundamental changes, there's a shift. If, as is unfortunately the case in more and more countries, a crucial maturation factor for the frontal lobe is missing—in our case, of course, the aquatic omega-3 fatty acids due to a Western diet—then a species-appropriate diet (green distribution) is inevitably replaced and leads to a leftward shift (red distribution) resulting in low or even very low performance.

This explains the dramatic increase in AD(H)D, autism, and disrupted social behavior. Of course, a lack of aquatic omega-3 fatty acids is only one of the factors responsible for such a development, because genuine social and economic reasons also play a role, but one should not ignore the contribution of nutritional physiology to neuropsychological and behavioral problems.

However, a general leftward shift in frontal lobe strength in the general population could also have contributed to the fact that our society as a whole has fundamentally changed in recent decades. An example of this is the ability to exert self-control that the frontal lobe gives us as part of its executive functions. For example, whether I eat the chocolate bar on the table in front of me in one go or whether my health is more important to me in the long term would be a decision that my frontal lobe has to make. A fundamental weakening of self-control in large parts of the population could explain why the short-term satisfaction of many supposed needs has become so important and dominates our way of life. The fast-food industry, for example, but also the IT, communications, and fashion industries are booming due to constantly growing consumerism. It is well known that these industries are anything but sustainable.

The widespread lack of self-control is, therefore, in complete contradiction to the actually deeply human need to give yourself and your own children and grandchildren the best possible future opportunities. The fact that the global consequences of a wasteful lifestyle are ignored also points to another function of the frontal lobe that could be disrupted by a general lack of aquatic omega-3 fatty acids: the ability to empathize. "Empathy plays a crucial

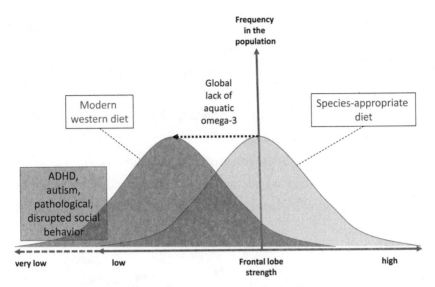

Change in normally distributed frontal lobe strength caused by a global lack of brain-building material due to a lack of aquatic omega-3 fatty acids.

interpersonal and social role, enables the exchange of experiences, needs, and wishes between individuals, and represents an emotional bridge, that promotes prosocial behavior," writes Helen Riess, doctor in the department for empathy and relational science at Harvard Medical School in Boston.[23]

All available empirical studies show that the decline in empathy is immense.[24] Empathic people are characterized by the basic ability to imagine the potential suffering they would inflict on others through certain actions. An increasing lack of empathy is typically accompanied by an increased tendency towards narcissism.[25] This is characterized by an exaggerated ego and sense of self-worth and thus an exaggerated tendency to put one's own well-being above that of others:[26] selfishness instead of altruism.

Increasing narcissism, coupled with an increasing loss of empathy, can also be seen at the political level. Right-wing populist parties are on the rise in almost all democracies. Even in Germany, the AfD and Pegida supporters are no longer marginal groups, despite the country's special past and intensive school education about the dangers of such a development. In the US, large parts of the population supported Donald Trump's "America first" approach, in view of the enormous global problems that the United States itself helped to cause and is still causing.

Trump's infamous Mexican wall project is perhaps the most obvious example of deliberate isolation and alienation from the

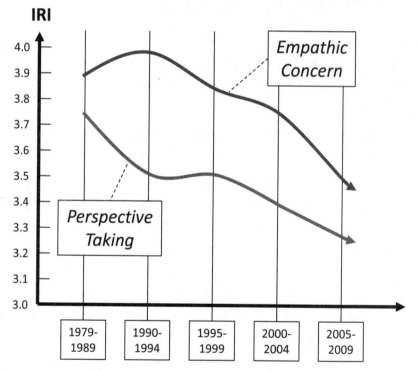

The ability to feel empathy decreases rapidly, as the International Reactivity Index (IRI) shows. A study with US college students over a period of thirty years (1979 to 2009) examined the ability to empathize with other people (Perspective Taking) or to feel sympathy for people in an unfortunate situation (Empathic Concern). The study result can be viewed as representative of Western society.

rest of the world. "Beware of America's shocking loss of empathy," writes human rights lawyer David Niose in *Psychology Today*.[27] He observes that this development is "unique in many ways." As an example, Niose cites Trump's public endorsement of using torture. In contrast to some of his predecessors, he did not even portray torture as a necessary evil.

Instead, he stressed at an election event: "Even if it doesn't work, they [the tortured] still deserve it." And his supporters broke out in cheers, as Niose reports. Trump was confident that the majority of American citizens who later elected him to the highest office expected such statements (and actions) from him.

Trump denigrates one group after another—Mexicans, Muslims, African Americans, Asians, women, and, of course, his competitors—and that is exactly how he increases his popularity. In Germany, with its own history marked by racism and xenophobia, the reaction is outraged, but at the same time hypocritical. Even representatives of bourgeois parties demand that foreigners should take a back seat when it comes to distributing food to those in need.[28] And the European counterpart to the "Mexican Wall" is located in the Mediterranean, just before the African mainland—and is no less inhumane. "At least 700 people drowned in the Mediterranean last week," *Der Spiegel* wrote the same year Trump scored points with the construction of the wall and continued: "But this hardly affects the Europeans anymore. They have gotten used to death at their borders."[29] Germans also have a "Germany or EU first" approach—we just don't say it out loud.

Science blames an increasing lack of empathy for the increasing destruction of the biosphere and biodiversity.[30] The extent of the worldwide destruction of species now is being compared

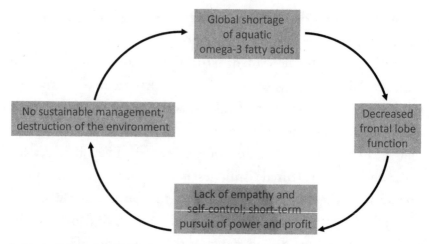

A vicious circle: a global lack of aquatic omega-3 fatty acids leads to global behaviors that exacerbate this global deficiency.

to that which destroyed not only the dinosaurs 65 million years ago, but over 90 percent of all life—but this time, the catastrophe is caused by humans. Gerardo Ceballos of the National Autonomous University of Mexico writes that "the massive loss of populations and species reflects our lack of compassion for all the wild species that have been our companions since our creation."[31] According to Ceballos, this is all just a prelude to the "decline of the natural systems that make our civilization possible." Think of the yeast fungi that do not have a frontal lobe and that destroy their habitat, and thus themselves, through unbridled growth. The vicious circle of self-destruction that humanity finds itself in is illustrated in the previous figure, as one of its causes could be a global shortage of aquatic omega-3 fatty acids.

Global challenges such as sustainably securing a species-appropriate world diet, ending progressive environmental destruction, as well as social justice and future opportunities for all people, require global solutions. Mastering this will only be possible with functioning frontal lobes that think and act socially and sustainably.[32] The previously quoted empathy researcher, Helen Riess, comes to the following conclusion in her article on the "Science of Empathy": "If we are to move in the direction of a more empathic society and a more compassionate world, it is clear that working to enhance our native capacities to empathize is critical to strengthening individual, community, national, and international bonds."[33]

To solve global problems, we need intelligent solutions (such as an efficient global supply of microalgae products), but interestingly, we do not necessarily need more rational intelligence—even if this would also increase with more aquatic omega-3 fatty acids. "Of course, intelligence is important in order to understand complex connections," said psychologist Tanja Gabriele Baudson in the science magazine *Spektrum*, "but what you ultimately do with this knowledge is a completely different argument, in which completely different personality traits come into play."[34] Intelligence, according to Baudson, does not protect against short-term selfish goals to prioritize sustainability over what is compatible with the common good and thus act ethically unacceptable. Emotional and social intelligence (EQ instead of IQ) is required to consider others' interests and do business sustainably for future generations.

If we fail to save the world and humanity from impending doom, each of us will have to take a good, long look at ourselves. In any case, blaming politics, economics, and capitalism for the destruction of our living space is too easy. There are no large systems or dark forces to blame. We decide for ourselves who we vote for, what we consume, or what profession we take up. All of our day-to-day decisions add up and have a global impact.

ALGAE OIL—
A FUTURE OPPORTUNITY
FOR ALL OF US

The lack of aquatic omega-3 fatty acids is a huge social problem. The average daily dose of around two grams that the new food algae oil currently provides (as of September 2024) costs around one dollar (US).[35] If all people were to demand their right to healthy development and the global community were to grant them this, sales would be around $7.5 billion daily or $2.737 billion per year—and thus 1.5 times that of the internet giant Google (as of September 2024).[36]

There would also be enough carbon dioxide for the photo-autotrophic production of algae oil, which could supply all of humanity with sufficient aquatic omega-3 fatty acids (and many other valuable raw materials).

My hope is that more and more people will recognize this unique opportunity to change something fundamentally, and that policy will set the course for more and more innovative companies to invest in the production of aquatic omega-3 fatty acids as a new food. As a result, the price on the free market would fall, especially if the valuable algae biomass is used across sectors. We could get to ten cents for a daily dose of essential omega-3 fatty acids, perhaps even significantly less. This means that everyone could afford it, and every person on our planet, whether young or old, would actually have the chance to live in a brain-friendly way and to exploit their intellectual potential. In this sense, the costs of global care could also be covered by the various savings in health care.

Microalgae indirectly provided a crucial building block for the development of the brain of modern humans and were, therefore, essential for their social conquest of the earth. Today, the direct use of microalgae could be indispensable for humanity's survival.

The loss of empathy and the increase in narcissism, depression, and anxiety in recent decades could therefore be explained by many changes in our way of life. But as complex as this mixture of causes and consequences may be, there is a very simple question:

How are you supposed to behave in a species-appropriate manner if you don't eat a species-appropriate diet?

Your personal response to this could be crucial.

GLOSSARY

AA—AA or Arachidonic Acid is a bioactive omega-6 fatty acid of animal origin; brain-building block, precursor of AA eicosanoids.

AA eicosanoids—a range of diverse hormonal substances derived from AA; biologically essential, but due to the modern Western diet, it is present in excess, and therefore AA eicosanoids are called the "bad" ones.

ALA—biologically inactive omega-3 fatty acid from land plants (therefore also referred to as terrestrial omega-3 fatty acid); ALA stands for alpha-linolenic acid; precursor of the bioactive omega-3 fatty acids EPA and DHA.

Aquatic Omega-3 Fatty Acids—EPA and DHA, which are primarily produced by microalgae and which enter the human diet via fish and seafood.

Bisphenol—toxic chemical products for plastic production.

Cis Fatty Acids—unsaturated fatty acids in a form that is natural for humans in contrast to trans fatty acids.

DHA—docosahexaenoic acid; a bioactive omega-3 fatty acid; brain-building block, precursor of DHA docosanoids.

DHA-Docosanoids—a range of diverse hormonal active ingredients formed from DHA; with generally positive health effects, therefore referred to as the "good ones."

EPA—eicosapentaenoic acid; bioactive omega-3 fatty acid; precursor of EPA eicosanoids and precursor of DHA.

EPA Eicosanoids—a range of diverse hormonal agents formed from EPA; with generally positive health effects, therefore referred to as the "good ones."

EPA and DHA—bioactive omega-3 fatty acids mainly formed by microalgae that reach us via the food chain from krill to fish and seafood, therefore referred to as aquatic omega-3 fatty acids, biologically active and beneficial to health.

F-Vitamins—historical term for the essential fatty acids ALA and LA, later expanded to EPA, DHA, and AA.

LA—Linoleic Acid, biologically inactive omega-6 fatty acid from land plants (therefore also referred to as terrestrial omega-6 fatty acid); precursor to AA.

Microalgae—single-celled organisms in fresh and salt water, part of plankton.

Omega-3 Fatty Acids—polyunsaturated, essential because our body cannot produce its basic structure itself; these include ALA, EPA, and DHA.

Omega-3 Index—percentage of aquatic omega-3 fatty acids EPA and DHA in relation to all fatty acids in the cell membrane of red blood cells.

Omega-6/3-Quotient (O-6/3-Q)—The relative ratio of omega-6 fatty acid AA to omega-3 fatty acid EPA, as measured in the red blood cell membrane.

Omega-6 Fatty Acids—Polyunsaturated, essential, because our body cannot produce this basic structure itself; these include LA and AA.

Omega-9 Fatty Acids—monounsaturated, not essential, as self-production possible; in the cis form known as oleic acid.

PCBs—polychlorinated biphenyls; chemical products, toxic.

PBDEs—Polybrominated diphenyl ethers; chemical products, toxic.

TBTs—Tributyltin or Tributyltin compounds; chemical products, toxic.

Trans Fatty Acids—unsaturated fatty acids in a form that is unnatural for humans and therefore unhealthy; in contrast to cis-fatty acids.

ACKNOWLEDGMENTS

My gratitude for the helpful comments and excellent suggestions to biologist Bettina Simonis, Dr. Med. Bernhard Dickreiter, Specialist in Internal Medicine, Physical Rehabilitative Medicine and Naturopathy, as well as the Microalgae Expert Peter Bergmann, MSc. Biotechnology, Head of Research and Development at Subitec LLC. Last but not least, I thank my wife, Sabine, once again for her tireless support.

REFERENCES

Bostrom, Nick: *Superintelligence: Paths, Dangers, Strategies*, New York: Oxford University Press 2014

Damasio, Antonio: *The Strange Order of Things: Life, Feeling, and the Making of Cultures*, New York: Pantheon 2018

Diamond, Jared: *The Rise and Fall of the Third Chimpanzee: Evolution and Human Life*, New York: Vintage 2003

Fukuoka, Masanobu: *The One-Straw Revolution: An Introduction to Natural Farming*, New York: Rodale Press 1978

Gøtzsche, Peter Christian: *Deadly Medicines and Organised Crime: How Big Pharma Has Corrupted Healthcare*, Boca Raton: CRC Press 2017

Harari, Yuval Noah: *Sapiens: A Brief History of Humankind*, New York: Harper 2015

Harari, Yuval Noah: *Homo Deus: A Brief History of Tomorrow*, New York: Harper 2017

Kopp, Thomas: *Auf Kosten Anderer? Wie die imperiale Lebensweise ein gutes Leben für alle verhindert*, München: Oekom 2017

Kurzweil, Ray: *The Singularity Is Near: When Humans Transcend Biology*, New York: Viking 2005

Kreiß, Christian: *Gekaufte Forschung: Wissenschaft im Dienst der Konzerne*, München: Europa 2015

Liebke, Frank: *Doktor Chlorella! Die Alge fürs Leben. Kompendium zur Mikroalge Chlorella*, Holm: RL-Verlagskontor 2007

Limberg, Axel: *Das Plankton-Manifest: Wie ein neuer Rohstoff die Welt verändern wird,* Hamburg: Zaunkönig 2007

Mau, Steffen: *The Metric Society: On the Quantification of the Social,* Cambridge: Polity 2019

Miegel, Meinhard: *Exit. Wohlstand ohne Wachstum,* Berlin: List 2012

Sapolsky, Robert: Behave: *The Biology of Humans at Our Best and Worst,* New York: Penguin Press 2017

Scheub, Ute, und Schwarzer, Stefan: *Die Humusrevolution. Wie wir den Boden heilen, das Klima retten und die Ernährungswende schaffen,* München: Oekom 2017

Shubin, Neil: *Your Inner Fish: A Journey into the 3.5-Billion-Year History of the Human Body,* New York: Pantheon 2008

Stiglitz, Joseph: *The Price of Inequality: How Today's Divided Society Endangers Our Future,* New York: W.W. Norton & Company 2012

Wilson, Edward Osborne: *The Social Conquest of Earth,* New York: W.W. Norton & Company 2012

ENDNOTES

PART I: THE EVOLUTION OF THE HUMAN MIND

1   Williams R: Microscopic algae produce half the oxygen we breathe. *The Science Show*. October 25, 2013. www.abc.net.au/radionational/programs/scienceshow/microscopic-algae-produce-half-the-oxygen-we-breathe/5041338.

2   Wiedmann TS et al: Lipid protein interactions mediate the photochemical function of rhodopsin. *Biochemistry* 1988, 27:6469–6474.

3   Fliesler SJ & Anderson RE: Chemistry and metabolism of lipids in the vertebrate retina. *Prog Lipid Res* 1983, 22:79–131.

4   Gawrisch K et al: The structure of DHA in phospholipid membranes. *Lipids* 2003, 38:445–452.

5   Mitchell DC & Litman BJ: Docosahexaenoic acid-containing phospholipids optimally promote rhodopsin activation. Essential Fatty Acids and Eicosanoids: Invited Papers from the Fourth International Congress. Champaign, American Oil Chemists' Society, 1998: 154–158.

6   Mihailescu M & Gawrisch K: The structure of polyunsaturated lipid bilayers important for rhodopsin function: A neutron diffraction study. *Biophys* 2006, 90:4–6.

7   Fliesler SJ & Anderson RE: Chemistry and metabolism of lipids in the vertebrate retina. *Prog Lipid Res* 1983,22:79–131.

8   Birch EE et al: Visual Acuity and the essentiality of docosahexaenoic acid and arachidonic acid in the diet of term infants. *Pediatr Res* 1998, 44:201–209.

9   Souied EH et al: Omega-3 Fatty Acids and Age-Related Macular Degeneration. *Ophthalmic Res* 2015, 55:62–69.

10 Tanaka K et al: Effects of docosahexaenoic acid on neurotransmission. *Bio-mol Ther* 2012, 20:152–157.

11 Bazan NG & Scott BL: Dietary omega-3 fatty acids and accumulation of docosahexaenoic acid in rod photoreceptor cells of the retina and at synapses. *UPS J Med Sci* Suppl 1990, 48:97–107.

12 Suzuki H et al: Rapid incorporation of docosahexaenoic acid from dietary sources into brain microsomal, synaptosomal and mitochondrial membrane in adult mice. *Int J Vitam Nutr* Res 1997, 67:272–278.

13 Crawford MA & Broadhurst CL: The role of docosahexaenoic and the marine food web as determinants of evolution and hominid brain development: The challenge for human sustainability. *Nutr Health* 2012, 21: 17–39.

14 Kawakita E et al: Docosahexaenoic acid promotes neurogenesis in vitro and in vivo. *Neuroscience* 2006, 139:991–997.

15 Koletzko B et al: The roles of long-chain polyunsaturated fatty acids in pregnancy, lactation, and infancy: Review of current knowledge and consensus recommendations. *J Perinat Med* 2008, 36:5–14.

16 Kang JX & Gleason ED: Omega-3 Fatty acids and hippocampal neurogenesis in depression. CNS *Neurol Disord Drug Targets* 2013, 12:460–465

17 Snyder JS et al: Adult hippocampal neurogenesis buffers stress responses and depressive behavior. *Nature* 2011, 476:458–461.

18 Nehls M: Unified theory of Alzheimer's disease (UTAD): Implications for prevention and curative therapy. *J Mol Psychiatry* 2016, www.ncbi. nlm.nih. GOV/PubMed/27429752.

19 Calderon F & Kim HY: Docosahexaenoic acid promotes neurite growth in hippocampal neurons. *J Neurochem* 2004, 90:979–988.

20 Zhao Y et al: Docosahexaenoic acid-derived neuroprotectin D1 induces neuronal survival via secretase- and PPARγ-mediated mechanisms in Alzheimer's disease models. PLoS One 2011, www.ncbi.nlm.nih.gov /PubMed/21246057; Asatryan A & Bazan NG: Molecular mechanisms of signaling via the docosanoid neuroprotectin D1 for cellular homeostasis and neuroprotection. *J Biol Chem* 2017, 292:12390–12397.

21 Michael-Titus AT & Priestley JV: Omega-3 fatty acids and traumatic neurological injury: From neuroprotection to neuroplasticity? *Trends Neurosci* 2014, 37:30–38.

22 Silva RV et al: Long-Chain Omega-3 Fatty Acids Supplementation Accelerates Nerve Regeneration and Prevents Neuropathic Pain Behavior

in Mice. *Front Pharmacol* 2017, www.ncbi.nlm.nih.gov/pubmed/290 89890.

23   Simón MV et al: Synthesis of docosahexaenoic acid from eicosapen-taenoic acid in retina neurons protects photoreceptors from oxidative stress. *J Neu-Rochem* 2016, 136:931–946.

24   Serhan CN: Pro-resolving lipid mediators are leads for resolution physi-ology. *Nature* 2014, 510:92–101.

25   Salem N Jr et al: Arachidonic and docosahexaenoic acids are biosynthe-sized from their 18-carbon precursors in human infants. *Proc Natl Acad Sci* USA 1996, 93:49–54.

26   Gibbons A: Humans' Head Start: New views of brain evolution. *Science* 2002, 296:835 ff.

27   Eaton SB & Konner M: Paleolithic Nutrition. A consideration of its nature and current implications. *N Engl J Med* 1985, 312: 283–289.

28   Crawford MA & Broadhurst CL: The role of docosahexaenoic and the marine food web as determinants of evolution and hominid brain devel-opment: The challenge for human sustainability. *Nutr Health* 2012, 21:17–39.

29   Ruff CB et al: Body mass and encephalization in Pleistocene Homo. *Nature* 1997, 387:173–176.

30   Behar DM et al: The Dawn of Human Matrilineal Diversity. *On J Hum Genet* 2008, 82:1130–1140.

31   Marean CW et al: Early human use of marine resources and pigment in South Africa during the Middle Pleistocene. *Nature* 2007, 449:905–908.

32   Marean CW et al: Als die Menschen fast ausstarben. *Spektrum der Wissenschaft* 2010, 12:59–65.

33   Orlich MJ et al: Vegetarian dietary patterns and mortality in Adventist Health Study 2. *JAMA Internal Med* 2013, 173:1230–1238.

34   Stetka B: By Land or by Sea: How Did Early Humans Access Key Brain-Building Nutrients? *Scientific American* 2016; www.scientificamerican .com/article/by-land-or-by-sea-how-did-early-humans-access-key-brain -building-nutrients

35   Brown KS et al: Fire as an engineering tool of early modern humans. *Science* 2009, 325:859–862.

36   Marean CW: The origins and significance of coastal resource use in Africa and Western Eurasia. *J Hum Evol* 2014, 77:17–40.

37   Bowles S: Did warfare among ancestral hunter-gatherers affect the evolution of human social behaviors? *Science* 2009, 324:1293–1298.

38   Hoffmann M: The human frontal lobes and frontal network systems: An evolutionary, clinical, and treatment perspective. *ISRN Neurol* 2013, www.ncbi.nlm.nih.gov/pubmed/23577266.

39   Bradbury J: Docosahexaenoic acid (DHA): An ancient nutrient for the modern human brain. *Nutrients* 2011, 3:529–554.

40   Boeckx C & Benítez-Burraco A: The shape of the human language-ready brain. *Front Psychol* 2014, www.ncbi.nlm.nih.gov/pubmed/24772099.

41   Bar-Yosef O: The role of western Asia in modern human origins. *Philos Trans R Soc Lond B Biol Sci* 1992, 337:193–20.

42   Strasser TF et al: Stone Age Seafaring in the Mediterranean: Evidence from the Plakias Region for Lower Palaeolithic and Mesolithic Habitation of Crete. *Hesperia* 2010, 79:145–190.

43   Richards MP et al: Isotope evidence for the intensive use of marine foods by Late Upper Palaeolithic humans. *J Hum Evol* 2005, 49:390–394.

44   Bocherens H et al: Isotopic evidence for diet and subsistence pattern of the Saint-Césaire I Neanderthal: Review and use of a multi-source mixing model. *J Hum Evol* 2005, 49:71–87.

45   Ruff CB et al: Body mass and encephalization in Pleistocene Homo. *Nature* 1997, 387:173–176.

46   Harari YN: A Brief History of Humankind. DVA 2013:101–125.

47   Figure adapted from: http://aquatic-human-ancestor.org/anatomy/brain.html.

48   Crabtree GR: Our fragile intellect. Part I & II. *Trends Genet* 2013, 29:1–5

49   Florio M et al: Human-specific genes ARHGAP11B promotes basal progenitor amplification and neocortex expansion. *Science* 2015 347: 1465–1470.

50   Shaffer J: Neuroplasticity and Clinical Practice: Building Brain Power for Health. *Front Psychol* 2016, www.ncbi.nlm.nih.gov/pubmed/27507957.

51   Kitajka K et al: Effects of dietary omega-3 polyunsaturated fatty acids on brain gene expression. *Proc Natl Acad Sci* USA 2004, 101:10931–10936.

52   Tan ZS et al: Red blood cell omega-3 fatty acid levels and markers of accelerated brain aging. *Neurology* 2012, 78:658–664; Pottala JV et al.: Higher RBC EPA + DHA corresponds with larger total brain and hippocampal volumes: WHIMS-MRI study. *Neurology* 2014, 82:435–442.

53 Kuipers RS et al: Estimated macronutrient and fatty acid intake from an East African Paleolithic diet. *BR J Nutr* 2010, 104:1666–1687.

PART II: AN EXCURSION INTO THE WORLD OF FATTY ACIDS

1 Kreiß C: Purchased Research—Science in the Service of Corporations. *Europa Verlag* 2015.

2 Orlich MJ et al: Vegetarian dietary patterns and mortality in Adventist Health Study 2. *JAMA Internal Med* 2013, 173:1230–1238; Michaëlsson K et al: Milk intake and risk of mortality and fractures in women and men: Cohort studies. *BMJ* 2014; www.ncbi.nlm.nih.gov/pmc/articles/PMC 4212225.

3 Tree SJ et al: Fatty acids in cardiovascular health and disease: A comprehensive update. J *Clin Lipidol* 2012, 6:216–234; Ramsden CE et al.: Re-evaluation of the traditional diet-heart hypothesis: Analysis of recovered data from Minnesota Coronary Experiment (1968–73.) *BMJ* 2016, www.ncbi.nlm.nih. GOV/PubMed/27071971.

4 Makki K et al: Obesity tissue in obesity-related inflammation and insulin resistance: Cells, cytokines, and chemokines. *ISRN Inflamm* 2013, www .NCBI. nlm.nih.gov/pubmed/24455420.

5 Gano LB et al: Ketogenic Diets, Mitochondria, and Neurological Diseases. *J Lipid Res* 2014, 55:2211–2228.

6 Grabacka M et al: Regulation of Ketone Body Metabolism and the Role of PPARα. *Int J Mol Sci* 2016, www.ncbi.nlm.nih.gov/pubmed/27983603.

7 Sleiman SF et al: Exercise promotes the expression of brain-derived neurotrophic factor (BDNF) through the action of the ketone body β-hydroxybutyrate. *ELife* 2016, www.ncbi.nlm.nih.gov/pubmed/2725 3067.

8 Burr GO & Burr MM: A new deficiency disease produced by rigid exclusion of fat from the diet. *J Biol Chem* 1929, 82: 345–336.

9 Smith W & Mukhopadhyay RJ: Essential fatty acids: The work of George and Mildred Burr. *Biol Chem* 2012, 287:35439–35441.

10 Bourre JM et al: Dietary alpha-linolenic acid at 1.3 g/kg maintains maximum docosahexaenoic acid concentration in brain, heart and liver of adult rats. *J Nutr* 1993, 123:1313–1319; Gao F et al: Quantifying conversion of linoleic to arachidonic and other n-6 polyunsaturated fatty acids in unanesthetized rats. *J Lipid Res* 2010, 51:2940–2946.

11 Goyens PL et al: Compartmental modeling to quantify alpha-linolenic acid conversion after longer term intake of multiple tracer boluses. *J Lipid Res* 2005, 46:1474–1483.

12 Hussein N et al: Long-chain conversion of [13C] linoleic acid and alpha-linolenic acid in response to marked changes in their dietary intake in men. *J Lipid Res* 2005, 46:269–280.

13 Gillingham LG et al: Dietary oils and FADS1-FADS2 genetic variants modulate [13C]α-linolenic acid metabolism and plasma fatty acid composition. *On J Clin Nutr* 2013, 97:195–207.

14 Baker EJ et al: Metabolism and functional effects of plant-derived omega-3 fatty acids in humans. *Prog Lipid Res* 2016, 64:30–56.

15 Lands B: Dietary omega-3 and omega-6 fatty acids compete in producing tissue compositions and tissue responses. *MIL Med* 2014, 179:76–81.

16 Salem N Jr et al: Arachidonic and docosahexaenoic acids are biosynthesized from their 18-carbon precursors in human infants. *Proc Natl Acad Sci* USA 1996, 93:49–54.

17 Harnack K et al: Quantitation of alpha-linolenic acid elongation to eicosapentaenoic and docosahexaenoic acid as affected by the ratio of n6/n3 fatty acids. *Nutr Metab* 2009, www.ncbi.nlm.nih.gov/pubmed /19228394.

18 Blasbalg TL et al: Changes in consumption of omega-3 and omega-6 fatty acids in the United States during the 20th Century. *On J Clin Nutr* 2011, 93:950–962.

19 Hibbeln JR et al: Healthy Intakes of n-3 and n-6 fatty acids: Estimations considering Worldwide Diversity. *On J Clin Nutr* 2006, 83: 1483–1493.

20 Simopoulos AP: Importance of the Omega-6/Omega-3 Balance in Health and Disease: Evolutionary aspects of diet. *World Rev Nutr Diet* 2011, 102:10–21.

21 Liou YA et al: Decreasing linoleic acid with constant alpha-linolenic acid in dietary fats increases (n-3) eicosapentaenoic acid in plasma phospholipids in healthy men. *J Nutr* 2007, 137:945–952.

22 Wood KE: The effect of modifying dietary LA and ALA Intakes on omega-3 long chain polyunsaturated fatty acid (n-3 LCPUFA) Status in human adults: A systematic review and commentary. *Prostaglandins Leukot. Essent Fat Acids* 2015, 95:47–55.

23 Okuyama H: Dietary fatty acids—The N-6/N-3 balance and chronic elderly diseases. Excess linoleic acid and relative N-3 deficiency syndrome lakes in Japan. *Prog Lipid Res* 1996, 35:409–457.

24 Grant WB: Trends in diet and Alzheimer's disease during the nutrition transition in Japan and developing countries. *J Alzheimers Dis* 2014, 38:611–620.

25 Kim H et al: Association between maternal intake of n-6 to n-3 fatty acid ratio during pregnancy and infant neurodevelopment at 6 months of age: Results of the MOCEH cohort study. *Nutr J* 2017, www.ncbi.nlm.nih .gov/PubMed/28420388.

26 McDougle DR et al: Anti-inflammatory omega-3 endocannabinoid epoxides. *Proc Natl Acad Sci* USA 2017, 114:6034–6043; Araque A et al: Synaptic functions of endocannabinoid signaling in health and disease. *Neuropharmacology* 2017, 124:13–24; Murillo-Rodriguez, E et al.: The emerging role of the endocannabinoid system in the sleep-wake cycle modulation. *Cent Nerv Syst Agents Med Chem* 2011, 11:189–196.

27 Dennis EA & Norris PC: Eicosanoid Storm in infection and inflammation. *Nat Rev Immunol* 2015, 15:511–523.

28 Shinohara M et al: Functional Metabolomics Reveals Novel Active Products in the DHA Metabolome. *Front Immunol* 2012, www.ncbi .nlm.nih.gov/PubMed/22566962.

29 Serhan CN et al: Protectins and maresins: New pro-resolving families of mediators in acute inflammation and resolution bioactive metabolome. *Biochim Biophys Acta* 2015, 1851:397–413.

30 Tokuda H et al: Differential effect of arachidonic acid and docosahexaenoic acid on age-related decreases in hippocampal neurogenesis. *Neurosci Res* 2014, 88:58–66.

31 Thomas MH et al: Dietary arachidonic acid as a risk factor for age-associated neurodegenerative diseases: Potential mechanisms. *Biochimie* 2016, 130: 168–177.

32 Asatryan A & Bazan NG: Molecular mechanisms of signaling via the docosanoid neuroprotectin D1 for cellular homeostasis and neuroprotection. *J Biol Chem* 2017, 292:12390–12397.

33 Das UN: Essential fatty acids and their metabolites could function as endogenous HMG-CoA reductase and ACE enzyme inhibitors, anti-arrhythmic, anti-hypertensive, anti-atherosclerotic, anti-inflammatory, cytoprotective, and cardioprotective molecules. *Lipids Health Dis* 2008, www.ncbi.nlm.nih. Gov/pmc/articles/PMC2576273.

34 Schuchardt JP & Hahn A: Bioavailability of long-chain omega-3 fatty acids. *Prostaglandins Leukot Essent Fatty Acids* 2013, 89:1–8.

35 www.omegametrix.eu.

36 von Schacky C & Harris WS: Cardiovascular benefits of omega-3 fatty acids. *Cardiovasc Res* 2007, 73:310–315; Harris WS: The Omega-3 index as a risk factor for coronary heart disease. *On J Clin Nutr* 2008, 87:1997–2002.

37 Martínez M & Mougan I: Fatty acid composition of human brain phospholipids during normal development. *J Neurochem* 1998, 71:2528–2533.

38 www.lgl.bayern.de/lebensmittel/warengruppen/wc_13_fette_oele/ ue_2007_ trans_fettsaeuren.htm.

39 Wallace SK & Mozaffarian D: Trans-fatty acids and nonlipid risk factors. *Curr Atheroscler Rep* 2009; www.ncbi.nlm.nih.gov/pubmed/19852883; Mozaf-Farian D et al: Health effects of trans-fatty acids: Experimental and observational evidence. *EUR J Clin Nutr* 2009, 63:5–21.

40 Sommerfeld M et al: Trans unsaturated fatty acids in natural products and processed foods. *Prog Lipid Res* 1983, 22:221–233; Pfalzgraf A et al.: Content of trans fatty acids in foods. *Z Ernährungswiss* 1993, 33:24–43

41 Laaninen, Tarja: Trans Fats—Overview of recent developments. Eurpean Union 2016; https://www.europarl.europa.eu/RegData/etudes/BRIE /2016/577966/EPRS_BRI(2016)577966_EN.pdf.

42 Nehls M: Kopfküche. *Das Anti-Alzheimer-Kochbuch: 50 unvergessliche Rezepte gegen Alzheimer & Co.* Systemed 2017.

43 Zárate J et al: A study of the toxic effect of oxidized sunflower oil containing 4-hydroperoxy-2-nonenal and 4-hydroxy-2-nonenal on cortical TrkA receptor expression in rats. *Nutr Neurosci* 2009, 12: 249–259; Gwon AR et al: "Oxidative lipid modification of nicastrin enhances amyloidogenic γ-secretase activity in Alzheimer's disease," *Aging Cell* 2012: 559–568; Di Domenico F et al: Role of 4-hydroxy-2-nonenal (HNE) in the pathogenesis of Alzheimer disease and other selected age-related neurodegenerative disorders. *Free Radic Biol Med* 2017, 111:253–261.

44 Sinclair HM. The diet of Canadian Eskimos. *Proc Nutr Soc* 1953, 12:69–82.

PART III: PANDEMICS DUE TO AQUATIC OMEGA-3 DEFICIENCY

1 Dobbing J & Sands J: Quantitative growth and development of human brain. *Arch Dis Child* 1973, 48:757–767.

2   Clandinin MT et al: Intrauterine fatty acid accretion rates in human brain: Implications for fatty acid requirements. *Early Hum Dev* 1980, 4:121–129.

3   Salem N Jr et al: Arachidonic and docosahexaenoic acids are biosynthesized from their 18-carbon precursors in human infants. *Proc Natl Acad Sci* USA 1996, 93:49–54.

4   Lauritzen L et al: The essentiality of long chain n-3 fatty acids in relation to development and function of the brain and retina. *Prog Lipid Res* 2001, 40:1–94.

5   Innis SM: Dietary omega 3 fatty acids and the developing brain. *Brain Research* 2008, 1237:35–43; Farquharson J et al.: Infant cerebral-cortex phospholipid fatty-acid composition and diet. *Lancet* 1992, 340:810–813; Grantham-McGregor S et al.: Developmental potential in the first 5 years for children in developing countries. *Lancet* 2007, 369:60–70.

6   Birch EE et al: Visual Acuity and cognitive outcomes at 4 years of age in a double-blind, randomized trial of long-chain polyunsaturated fatty acid-supplemented infant formula. *Early Hum Dev* 2007, 83:279–284.

7   Burdge GC & Wootton SA: Conversion of alpha-linolenic acid to eicosapaftaenoic, docosapentaenoic and docosahexaenoic acids in young women. *BR J Nutr* 2002; 88:411-420; Burdge GC: Eicosapentaenoic and docosapentaenoic acids are the principal products of alpha-linolenic acid metabolism in young men. *BR J Nutr* 2002;88:355–363.

8   Francois CA et al: Supplementing lactating women with flaxseed oil does not increase docosahexaenoic acid in their milk. *On J Clin Nutr* 2003, 77:226–733.

9   Brenna JT et al: Alpha-linolenic acid supplementation and conversion to n-3 long-chain polyunsaturated fatty acids in humans. *Prostaglandins Leukot Essent Fatty Acids* 2009, 80:85–91.

10   Cunnane SC et al: Breast-fed infants achieve a higher rate of brain and whole body docosahexaenoate accumulation than formula-fed infants not consuming dietary docosahexaenoate. *Lipids* 2000, 35:105–111.

11   Pittet PG et al: Site differences in the fatty acid composition of subcutaneous adipose tissue of obese women. *BR J Nutr* 1979, 42:57–61; Malcom GT et al: Fatty acid composition of adipose tissue in humans: Differences between subcutaneous sites. *On J Clin Nutr* 1989, 50:288–291.

12 Singh D et al: Did the perils of abdominal obesity affect depiction of feminine beauty in the sixteenth to eighteenth century British literature? Exploring the health and beauty link. *Proc Biol Sci* 2007, 274:891–894.

13 Storck Lindholm E et al: Different fatty acid pattern in breast milk of obese compared to normal-weight mothers. *Prostaglandins Leukot Essent Fatty Acids* 2013, 88:211–217.

14 Lasseka WD & Gaulin SJC: Waist-hip ratio and cognitive ability: Is gluteofemoral fat a privileged store of neurodevelopmental resources? *Evolution and Human Behavior* 2008, 29:26–34.

15 Lassek WD & Gaulin SJ: Changes in body fat distribution in relation to parity in American Women: A cover form of maternal depletion. *Am J Phys Anthropol* 2006, 131:295–302.

16 Butovskaya M et al: Waist-to-hip ratio, body-mass index, age and number of children in seven traditional societies. *SCI Rep* 2017, www.ncbi. nlm.nih.gov/PMC/articles/PMC5431669.

17 Bourre JM: Dietary omega-3 fatty acids for women. *Biomed Pharmacother* 2007, 61:105–112.

18 Brenna JT et al: Docosahexaenoic and arachidonic acid concentrations in human breast milk worldwide. *On J Clin Nutr* 2007, 85:1457–1464.

19 Del Prado M et al: Contribution of dietary and newly formed arachidonic acid to human milk lipids in women eating a low-fat diet. *On J Clin Nutr* 2001, 74:242–247.

20 Oken E et al: Associations of maternal fish intake during pregnancy and breastfeeding duration with attainment of developmental milestones in early childhood: A study from the Danish National Birth Cohort. *The American Journal of Clinical Nutrition*. 2008, 88:789–796.

21 Helland IB et al: Maternal supplementation with very-long-chain n-3 fatty acids during pregnancy and lactation augments children's IQ at 4 years of age. *Pediatrics* 2003, 111:39–44.

22 Dunstan JA et al: Cognitive assessment of children at age 2(1/2) years after maternal fish oil supplementation in pregnancy: A randomized controlled trial. *Arch Dis Child Fetal Neonatal Ed* 2008, 93:45–50; Jensen CL et al.: Effects of maternal docosahexaenoic acid intake on visual function and neuro-development in breastfed term infants. *On J Clin Nutr* 2005, 82:125–132.

23 Ramakrishnan U et al: Effects of docosahexaenoic acid supplementation during pregnancy on gestational age and size at birth: Randomized, double-blind, placebo-controlled trial in Mexico. *Food Nutr Bull* 2010, 31:108–116.

24 Veena SR et al: Association of birth weight and head circumference at birth to cognitive performance in 9–10-year-old children in South India: Prospective birth cohort study. *Pediatr Res* 2010, 67: 424–429.

25 Boucher O et al.: Neurophysiologic and neurobehavioral evidence of beneficial effects of prenatal omega-3 fatty acid intake on memory function at school age. *On J Clin Nutr* 2011, 93:1025–1037.

26 Cohen JT et al: A quantitative analysis of prenatal intake of n-3 polyunsaturated fatty acids and cognitive development. *On J Prev Med* 2005, 29:366–374.

27 Helland IB et al: Effect of supplementing pregnant and lactating mothers with n-3 very-long-chain fatty acids on children's IQ and body mass index at 7 years of age. *Pediatrics* 2008, 122:472–479.

28 Lassek WD, Gaulin, SJC: Linoleic and docosahexaenoic acids in human milk have opposite relationships with cognitive test performance in a sample of 28 countries. *Prostaglandins Leukot Essent Fatty Acids* 2014; 91:195–201.

29 Blencowe H et al: Born Too Soon: The global epidemiology of 15 million preterm births. *Reprod Health* 2013, www.ncbi.nlm.nih.gov/pmc/articles/PMC3828585.

30 Baack ML et al: Long-chain polyunsaturated fatty acid levels in US donor human milk: Meeting the needs of premature infants? *J Perinatol* 2012, 32:598–603.

31 Baack ML et al: What is the relationship between gestational age and doco-sahexaenoic acid (DHA) and arachidonic acid (ARA) levels? *Prostaglandins Leukot Essent Fat Acids* 2015, 100:5–11.

32 De Rooy L et al: Extremely preterm infants receiving standard care receive very low levels of arachidonic and docosahexaenoic acids. *Clin Nutr* 2016; www.ncbi.nlm.nih.gov/pubmed/27756480.

33 Henriksen C et al: Improved cognitive development among preterm infants attributable to early supplementation of human milk with docosahexaenoic acid and arachidonic acid. *Pediatrics.* 2008, 121:1137–1145.

34 Davidoff MJ et al: Changes in the gestational age distribution among U.S. singleton births: Impact on rates of late preterm birth, 1992 to 2002. *Semin Perinatol* 2006, 30:8–15.

35 Greenberg JA et al: Omega-3 fatty acid supplementation during pregnancy. *Rev Obst Gynecol* 2008, 1:162–169; Olsen, S.F., Sorensen JD et al: Randomized controlled trial of effect of fish-oil supplementation on pregnancy duration. *Lancet* 1992, 339:1003–1007.

36 Kar S et al: Effects of omega-3 fatty acids in prevention of early preterm delivery: A systematic review and meta-analysis of randomized studies. *EUR J Gynecol Reprod Biol* 2016, 198:40–46.

37 Murray SR et al: Long term cognitive outcomes of early term (37–38 weeks) and late preterm (34–36 weeks) births: A systematic review. *Wellcome Open Res* 2017, www.ncbi.nlm.nih.gov/pmc/articles/PMC5721566.

38 Shireman TI et al: Docosahexaenoic acid supplementation (DHA) and the return on investment for pregnancy outcomes. *Prostaglandins Leukot Essent Fat Acids* 2016, 111:8–10.

39 Vannucci RC et al: Frontal lobe expansion during development using MRI and endocasts: Relation to microcephaly and homo floresiensis. *Anat Rec* 2013, 296: 630–637.

40 Hill J et al: Similar Patterns of cortical expansion during human development and evolution. *Proc Natl Acad Sci* USA 2010, 107:13135–13140.

41 Adapted from: Martínez M & Mougan I: Fatty acid composition of human brain phospholipids during normal development. *J Neurochem* 1998, 71:2528–2533.

42 Hilger K et al: Intelligence is associated with the modular structure of intrinsic brain networks. *SCI Rep* 2017, www.ncbi.nlm.nih.gov/pmc/articles/PMC5700184.

43 Brown TT & Jernigan TL: Brain development during the preschool years. *Neuropsychol Rev* 2012, 22:313–333

44 Macadam PS & Dettwyler KA: *Breastfeeding: Biocultural Perspectives.* Transaction Publishers 1995.

45 Barkley RA: The executive functions and self-regulation: An evolutionary neuropsychological perspective. *Neuropsychol Rev* 2001, 11:1–29; Anderson V et al: Attentional skills following traumatic brain injury in childhood: A component analysis. *Brain Inj* 1998, 12:937–949.

46 Barkley RA: The executive functions and self-regulation: An evolutionary neuropsychological perspective. *Neuropsychol Rev* 2001, 11:1–29; Steinberg L: Psychological Control: Style or substance? *New Dir Child Adolesc Dev* 2005, 108:71–78.

47 Gałecki P & Talarowska M: The Evolutionary Theory of Depression. *Med Sci Monit* 2017, 23:2267–2274.

48 Hart SL et al: Brief report: Newborn behavior differs with decosahexaenoic acid levels in breast milk. *J Pediatr Psychol* 2006, 31:221–226.

49 Mulder KA et al: Omega-3 fatty acid deficiency in infants before birth identified using a randomized trial of maternal DHA supplementation in pregnancy. *PLoS One* 2014, www.ncbi.nlm.nih.gov/pmc/articles/PMC 3888379.

50 Colombo J et al: Maternal DHA and the development of attention in infancy and toddlerhood. *Child Dev* 2004, 75:1254–1267; Jensen CL et al: Effects of early maternal docosahexaenoic acid intake on neuropsychological status and visual acuity at five years of age of breast-fed term infants. *J Pediatr* 2010, 157:900–905.

51 Boucher O et al: Neurophysiologic and neurobehavioral evidence of beneficial effects of prenatal omega-3 fatty acid intake on memory function at school age. *Am J Clin Nutr* 2011, 93:1025–1037.

52 Hibbeln JR et al: Maternal seafood consumption in pregnancy and neuro-developmental outcomes in childhood (ALSPAC study): an observational cohort study. *Lancet* 2007, 369:578–585.

53 McNamara RK et al: Docosahexaenoic acid supplementation increases prefrontal cortex activation during sustained attention in healthy boys: A placebo-controlled, dose-ranging, functional magnetic resonance imaging study. *Am J Clin Nutr* 2010, 91:1060–1067; Boucher O et al: Neurophysiologic and neurobehavioral evidence of beneficial effects of prenatal omega-3 fatty acid intake on memory function at school age. *Am J Clin Nutr* 2011, 93: 1025–1037; Jackson PA et al: Docosahexaenoic acid-rich fish oil modulates the cerebral hemodynamic response to cognitive tasks in healthy young adults. *Biol Psychol* 2012, 89:183–190.

54 Richardson AJ et al: Docosahexaenoic acid for reading, cognition and behavior in children aged 7–9 years: A randomized, controlled trial (the DOLAB Study.) *PLoS One* 2012, www.ncbi.nlm.nih.gov /pubmed/22970149.

55 Dalton A et al: A randomised control trial in schoolchildren showed improvement in cognitive function after consuming a bread spread, containing fish flour from a marine source. *Prostaglandins Leukot Essent Fatty Acids* 2009, 80:143–149.

56 Portillo-Reyes V et al: Clinical significance of neuropsychological improvement after supplementation with omega-3 in 8–12 years old malnourished Mexican children: a randomized, double-blind, placebo and treatment clinical trial. *Res Dev Disabil* 2014, 35:861–870.

57 Liu J et al: The mediating role of sleep in the fish consumption— cognitive functioning relationship: a cohort study. *Sci Rep* 2017, www.ncbi.nlm.nih. gov/pubmed/29269884.

58 Pusceddu MM et al: N-3 Polyunsaturated Fatty Acids through the Lifespan: Implication for Psychopathology. *Int J Neuropsychopharmacol* 2016, www.ncbi.nlm.nih.gov/pmc/articles/PMC5203760.

59 Kim SW et al: Relationship between Erythrocyte Fatty Acid Composition and Psycho-pathology in the Vienna Omega-3 Study. *PLoS One* 2016, www.ncbi.nlm.nih.gov/pmc/articles/PMC4786267.

60 Franke B et al: The genetics of attention deficit/hyperactivity disorder in adults, a review. *Mol Psychiatry* 2012, 17:960–987.

61 Asherson P et al: Adult attention-deficit hyperactivity disorder: key conceptual issues. *Lancet Psychiatry* 2016, 3:568–578.

62 Gray C & Climie EA: Children with Attention Deficit/Hyperactivity Disorder and Reading Disability: A Review of the Efficacy of Medication Treatments. *Front Psychol* 2016, www.ncbi.nlm.nih.gov/pmc/articles/PMC 4932103.

63 Burleson W: A Review of Co-Morbid Depression in Pediatric ADHD: Etiologies, Phenomenology, and Treatment. *J Child Adolesc Psychopharmacol* 2008, 18: 565–571.

64 Angold A et al: Co-morbidity. *J Child Psychol Psychiatry* 1999, 40:57–87.

65 Young Xia W et al: Comorbid anxiety and depression in school-aged children with attention deficit hyperactivity disorder (ADHD) and self-reported symptoms of ADHD, anxiety, and depression among parents of school-aged children with and without ADHD. *Shanghai Arch Psychiatry* 2015, 27:356–367.

66 Yang TX et al: Impaired Memory for Instructions in Children with Attention-Deficit Hyperactivity Disorder Is Improved by Action at

Presentation and Recall. *Front Psychol* 2017, www.ncbi.nlm.nih.gov/pmc /articles/PMC5258743.

67 Alchanatis M et al: Frontal brain lobe impairment in obstructive sleep apnea: A proton MR spectroscopy study. *EUR Respir J* 2004, 24980–986.

68 Liu J et al: The mediating role of sleep in the fish consumption— cognitive functioning relationship: a cohort study. *Sci Rep* 2017, www .ncbi.nlm.nih. gov/pubmed/29269884.

69 Hawkey E & Nigg JT: Omega-3 fatty acid and ADHD: blood level analysis and meta-analytic extension of supplementation trials. *Clin Psychol Rev* 2014, 34:496–505.

70 Milte CM et al: Eicosapentaenoic and docosahexaenoic acids, cognition, and behavior in children with attention-deficit/hyperactivity disorder: A randomized controlled trial. *Nutrition* 2012, 28:670–677.

71 Derbyshire E: Do Omega-3/6 Fatty Acids Have a Therapeutic Role in Children and Young People with ADHD? *J Lipids* 2017, www.ncbi.nlm .nih. Gov/pmc/articles/PMC5603098.

72 Woo HD et al: Dietary patterns in children with attention deficit /hyper-activity disorder (ADHD.) *Nutrients* 2014, 6:1539–1553.

73 Sharif MR et al: The Relationship between Serum Vitamin D Level and Attention Deficit Hyperactivity Disorder. *Iran J Child Neurol* 2015, 9: 48–53.

74 Spikins P: How our autistic ancestors played an important role in human evolution. *The Conversation* 2017, https://theconversation.com/how -our-autistic-ancestors-played-an-important-role-in-human-evolution -73477.

75 Fombonne E: Epidemiology of pervasive developmental disorders. *Pediatr Res* 2009, 65:591–598.

76 Van Elst K et al: Food for thought: Dietary changes in essential fatty acid ratios and the increase in autism spectrum disorders. *Neurosci Biobehav Rev* 2014, 45:369–378.

77 Chen J et al: Synaptic proteins and receptors defects in autism spectrum disorders. *Front Cell Neurosci* 2014, www.ncbi.nlm.nih.gov/pmc/articles /PMC4161164.

78 James S et al: Omega-3 fatty acids supplementation for autism spectrum disorders (ASD.) *Cochrane Database Syst Rev* 2011, www.ncbi.nlm.nih . GOV/PubMed/22071839.

79 Meguid NA et al: Role of polyunsaturated fatty acids in the management of Egyptian children with autism. *Clin Biochem* 2008, 41:1044–1048.

80 Kinney DK et al: Relation of schizophrenia prevalence to Latitude, Climate, fish consumption, infant mortality, and skin color: A role for prenatal vitamin d deficiency and infections? *Schizophr Bull* 2009, 35:582–595.

81 Pawełczyk T et al: Omega-3 fatty acid supplementation may prevent loss of gray matter thickness in the left parieto-occipital cortex in first episode schizophrenia: A secondary outcome analysis of the OFFER randomized controlled study. *Schizophr Res* 2017, www.ncbi.nlm.nih. GOV /PubMed/29079060.

82 Mossaheb N et al: Polyunsaturated fatty acids in emerging psychosis. *Curr Pharm Des* 2012, 18:576–591.

83 Amminger GP et al: Long-chain omega-3 fatty acids for indicated prevention of psychotic disorders: a randomized, placebo-controlled trial. *Arch Gen Psychiatry* 2010, 67:146–154.

84 Amminger GP et al: Longer-term outcome in the prevention of psychotic disorders by the Vienna Omega-3 study. *Nature Communications* 2015, www. nature.com/articles/ncomms8934.pdf.

85 Hensch TK: Critical period plasticity in local cortical circuits. *Nat Rev Neurosci* 2005, 6:877–888; Arain M et al: Maturation of the adolescent brain. *Neuropsychiatr Dis Treat* 2013, 9:449–461.

86 Patrick RP & Ames BN: Vitamin D and the omega-3 fatty acids control serotonin synthesis and action, part 2: relevance for ADHD, bipolar disorder, schizophrenia, and impulsive behavior. *FASEB J* 2015, 29:2207–2222.

87 Gałecki P & Talarowska M: The Evolutionary Theory of Depression. *Med Sci Monit* 2017, 23:2267–2274; Snyder JS et al: Adult hippocampal neurogenesis buffers stress responses and depressive behaviour. *Nature* 2011, 476:458–461; Hill AS et al: Increasing Adult Hippocampal Neurogenesis is Sufficient to Reduce Anxiety and Depression-Like Behaviors. *Neuropsychopharmacology* 2015, 40:2368–2378.

88 Spalding KL et al: Dynamics of hippocampal neurogenesis in adult humans. *Cell* 2013, 153:1219–1227.

89 Ryu JR et al: Control of adult neurogenesis by programmed cell death in the mammalian brain. *Mol Brain* 2016, www.ncbi.nlm.nih.gov/pmc

/articles/PMC4839132; Lin YT et al: Oxytocin stimulates hippocampal neurogenesis via oxytocin receptor expressed in CA3 pyramidal neurons. *Nat Commun* 2017, www.ncbi.nlm.nih.gov/pmc/articles/PMC5599651.

90 Su K-P et al.: Omega-3 Polyunsaturated Fatty Acids in Prevention of Mood and Anxiety Disorders. *Clin Psychopharmacol Neurosci* 2015, 13:129–137.

91 Golding J et al: High levels of depressive symptoms in pregnancy with low omega-3 fatty acid intake from fish. *Epidemiology* 2009, 20:598–603.

92 Markhus MW et al: Low Omega-3 index in pregnancy is a possible biological risk factor for postpartum depression. *PLoS One* 2013, www.ncbi.nlm.nih. Gov/pmc/articles/PMC3701051.

93 Monk C: Stress and mood disorders during pregnancy: Implications for child development. *Psychiatr Quarterly* 2001, 72:347–357.

94 Coletta JM et al: Omega-3 Fatty Acids and Pregnancy. *Rev Obst Gynecol* 2010, 3: 163–171.

95 Kaviani M et al: The Effect of Omega-3 Fatty Acid Supplementation on Maternal Depression during Pregnancy: A Double Blind Randomized Controlled Clinical Trial. *Int J Community Based Nurs Midwifery* 2014, 2:142–147; Makrides M et al: Effect of DHA supplementation during pregnancy on maternal depression and neurodevelopment of young children: a randomized controlled trial. *JAMA* 2010, 304:1675–1683; Su KP et al: Omega-3 fatty acids for major depressive disorder during pregnancy: Results from a randomized, double-blind, placebo-controlled trial. *J Clin Psychiatry* 2008, 69:644–651.

96 Hibbeln JR et al: Fish consumption and major depression. *Lancet* 1998, 351:1213.

97 Nemets H et al: Omega-3 Treatment of childhood depression: A controlled, double-blind pilot study. *Am J Psychiatry* 2006, 163:1098–1100.

98 Nehls M: Unified theory of Alzheimer's disease (UTAD): Implications for prevention and curative therapy. *J Mol Psychiatry* 2016, www.ncbi.nlm.nih. Gov/pmc/articles/PMC4947325.

99 Stonehouse W: Does Consumption of LC Omega-3 PUFA Enhance Cognitive Performance in Healthy School-Aged Children and throughout Adulthood? Evidence from Clinical Trials. *Nutrients* 2014, 6: 2730–2758; Bhatia HS et al: Omega-3 fatty acid deficiency during brain maturation reduces neuronal and behavioral plasticity in adulthood. *PLoS One* 2011, www.ncbi.nlm.nih.gov/PMC/articles/PMC3233581.

100 Klein RG et al: Clinical and functional outcome of childhood attention-deficit/hyperactivity disorder 33 years later. *Arch Gen Psychiatry* 2012, 69:1295–1303.

101 Gottfredson LS & Deary IJ: Intelligence Predicts Health and Longevity, but Why? *Curr Dir Psychol* 2004, 13:1–4.

102 Morrison F & Cosden M: Risk, resilience, and adjustment of individuals with learning disabilities. *Learn Disabil Q* 1997, 20:43–60.

103 Armbruster B et al: Putting Reading First. In The Research Building Blocks for Teaching Children to Read: Kindergarten through Grade 3, 3rd ed.; Adler, R., Ed.; Diane Publishing Co.: Darby, PA, USA, 2010.

104 Snow C et al: *Preventing Reading Difficulties in Young Children.* National Academies Press: Washington, DC, USA, 1998.

105 Nehls M: Unified theory of Alzheimer's disease (UTAD): Implications for prevention and curative therapy. *J Mol Psychiatry* 2016, www.ncbi.nlm.nih. Gov/pmc/articles/PMC4947325.

106 Conquer JA et al: Fatty acid analysis of blood plasma of patients with Alzheimer's disease, other types of dementia, and cognitive impairment. *Lipids* 2000, 35:1305–1312; Lin PY et al.: A meta-analytical review of polyunsaturated fatty acid compositions in dementia. *J Clin Psychiatry* 2012, 73:1245–1254; Schaefer et al: Plasma phosphatidylcholine docosahexaenoic acid content and risk of dementia and Alzheimer disease: The Framingham Heart Study. *Arch Neurol* 2006, 63:1545–1550.

107 Eriksdotter M et al: Plasma Fatty Acid Profiles in Relation to Cognition and Gender in Alzheimer's Disease Patients During Oral Omega-3 Fatty Acid Supplementation: The OmegAD Study. *J Alzheimers Dis* 2015, 48:805–812; Famenini S et al: Increased intermediate M1-M2 macrophage polarization and improved cognition in mild cognitive impairment patients on ω-3 supplementation. *FASEB J* 2017, 31:148–160; Yurko-Mauro K et al: Docosahexaenoic acid and adult memory: a systematic review and meta-analysis. *PLoS ONE* 2015, www.ncbi.nlm.nih .gov/pmc/articles/PMC4364972.

108 Belkouch M et al: The pleiotropic effects of omega-3 docosahexaenoic acid on the hallmarks of Alzheimer's disease. *J Nutr Biochem* 2016, 38:1–11; Asatryan A & Bazan NG: Molecular mechanisms of signaling via the docosanoid neuroprotectin D1 for cellular homeostasis and neuroprotection. *J Biol Chem* 2017, 292:12390–12397.

109 Zhao Y et al: Docosahexaenoic acid-derived neuroprotectin D1 induces neuronal survival via secretase- and PPARγ-mediated mechanisms in Alzheimer's disease models. *PLoS One* 2011, www.ncbi.nlm.nih.gov /pmc/articles/PMC3016440.

110 Bazan NG: The docosanoid neuroprotectin D1 induces homeostatic regulation of neuroinflammation and cell survival. *Prostaglandins Leukot Essent Fatty Acids* 2013, 88:127–179.

111 Yassine HN et al: Association of Serum Docosahexaenoic Acid With Cerebral Amyloidosis. *JAMA Neurol* 2016, 73:1208–1216.

112 Agrawal R & Gomez-Pinilla F: Metabolic syndrome in the brain: deficiency in omega-3 fatty acid exacerbates dysfunctions in insulin receptor signalling and cognition. *J Physiol* 2012, 590:2485–2499.

113 Nehls M: Die Alzheimer-Lüge—Die Wahrheit über eine vermeidbare Krankheit. Heyne 2014.

114 Nehls M: *Alzheimer ist heilbar—Rechtzeitig zurück in ein gesundes Leben.* Heyne 2015; Nehls M: *Die Formel gegen Alzheimer.* Heyne 2018; Braszus M: Therapien gegen das große Vergessen. Was hilft bei Alzheimer? SWR2 21.9.2017, www.swr.de/swr2/programm/sendungen/wissen/alzheimer -stand/-/id=660374/did=17944114/nid=660374/4hadoa/index.html.

115 Maiti P et al: Current understanding of the molecular mechanisms in Parkinson's disease: Targets for potential treatments. *Transl Neurodegener* 2017, www.ncbi.nlm.nih.gov/pmc/articles/PMC5655877.

116 Bridi JC & Hirth F: Mechanisms of α-Synuclein Induced Synaptopathy in Parkinson's Disease. *Front Neurosci* 2018, www.ncbi.nlm.nih.gov/pmc /articles/PMC5825910.

117 Seidl SE et al: The emerging role of nutrition in Parkinson's disease. *Front Aging Neurosci* 2014, www.ncbi.nlm.nih.gov/pmc/articles/PMC3945400.

118 Romano A et al: Linking lipid peroxidation and neuropsychiatric disorders: focus on 4-hydroxy-2-nonenal. *Free Radic Biol Med* 2017, 111:281–293.

119 Mischley LK et al: Role of Diet and Nutritional Supplements in Parkinson's Disease Progression. *Oxid Med Cell Longev* 2017, www.ncbi .nlm.nih.gov/pmc/articles/PMC5610862 nih.gov/pmc/articles/PMC56 10862www.ncbi. nlm.nih.gov/pmc/articles/PMC5610862.

120 Fabelo N et al: Severe alterations in lipid composition of frontal cortex lipid rafts from Parkinson's disease and incidental Parkinson's disease. *Mol Med* 2011, 17:1107–1118.

121 Mischley LK et al: Role of Diet and Nutritional Supplements in Parkinson's Disease Progression. *Oxid Med Cell Longev* 2017, www.ncbi .nlm.nih.gov/pmc/articles/PMC5610862 nih.gov/pmc/articles/PMC5610 862www.ncbi. nlm.nih.gov/pmc/articles/PMC5610862.

122 Michael-Titus AT & Priestley JV: Omega-3 fatty acids and traumatic neurological injury: From neuroprotection to neuroplasticity? *Trends Neurosci* 2014, 37:30–38; Chen X et al: Omega-3 polyunsaturated fatty acid supplementation attenuates microglial-induced inflammation by inhibiting the HMGB1/TLR4/NF-κB pathway following experimental traumatic brain injury. *J Neuroinflammation* 2017, www.ncbi.nlm.nih .gov/pmc/articles/PMC5525354.

123 Haar CV et al: Vitamins and nutrients as primary treatments in experimental brain injury: Clinical implications for nutraceutical therapies. *Brain Res* 2016, 1640:114–129.

124 Bang HO et al: The composition of the Eskimo food in north western Greenland. *Am J Clin Nutr* 1980, 33:2657–2661.

125 Sinclair HM: Deficiency of essential fatty acids and atherosclerosis, etcetera. *Lancet* 1956, 270:381–383.

126 Sinclair HM: Advantages and disadvantages of an Eskimo diet. Drugs Affecting Lipid Metabolism. Amsterdam: Elsevier/North-Holland Biomedical Press 1980, 363–370.

127 Kromhout D et al: Fish oil and omega-3 fatty acids in cardiovascular disease: do they really work? *Eur Heart J* 2012, 33: 436–443.

128 Ander BP et al.: Polyunsaturated fatty acids and their effects on cardiovascular disease. *Exp Clin Cardiol* 2003, 8: 164–172.

129 Capó X et al: Resolvins as proresolving inflammatory mediators in cardiovascular disease. *Eur J Med Chem* 2017, www.ncbi.nlm.nih.gov /pubmed/28732558; Fredman G & Tabas I: Boosting Inflammation Resolution in Atherosclerosis: The Next Frontier for Therapy. *Am J Pathol* 2017, 187:1211–1221.

130 Harris WS: The omega-3 index as a risk factor for coronary heart disease. *Am J Clin Nutr* 2008, 87:1997–2002; von Schacky C: Omega-3 Index and Cardiovascular Health. *Nutrients* 2014, 6: 799–814.

131 Calzolari I et al: Polyunsaturated fatty acids and cardiovascular disease. *Curr Pharm Des* 2009, 15:4094–4102; Fuhrmann W: Reduktion des plötzlichen Herztodes durch Omega-3-Fettsäuren in der Sekundärprävention des Myokardinfarktes. *Austrian Journal of Cardiology* 2003, 10: 504–508.

132 Micha R et al: Mozaffarian, D. Association Between Dietary Factors and Mortality From Heart Disease, Stroke, and Type 2 Diabetes in the United States. *JAMA* 2017, 317:912–924.

133 Rommelfanger J: Fischöl floppt erneut in der kardiovaskulären Risikoprävention. *Medscape* 17.3.2013, https://deutsch.medscape.com /artikel/4901083.

134 Saber H et al: Omega-3 Fatty Acids and Incident Ischemic Stroke and Its Atherothrombotic and Cardioembolic Subtypes in 3 US Cohorts. *Stroke* 2017, 48:2678–2685.

135 Kuszewski JC et al: Effects of Long-Chain Omega-3 Polyunsaturated Fatty Acids on Endothelial Vasodilator Function and Cognition-Are They Interrelated? *Nutrients* 2017, www.ncbi.nlm.nih.gov/pmc/articles /PMC5452217.

136 Mozaffarian D & Wu JH: (N-3) fatty acids and cardiovascular health: Are effects of EPA and DHA shared or complementary? *J Nutr* 2012, 142:614–625.

137 GBD 2015 Obesity Collaborators et al.: Health Effects of Overweight and Obesity in 195 Countries over 25 Years. *N Engl J Med* 2017, 377:13–27.

138 Simopoulos AP: An Increase in the Omega-6/Omega-3 Fatty Acid Ratio Increases the Risk for Obesity. *Nutrients* 2016, www.ncbi.nlm.nih.gov /pmc/articles/PMC4808858.

139 Amri EZ et al: Fatty acids as signal transducing molecules: Involvement in the differentiation of preadipose to adipose cells. *J Lipid Res* 1994, 35:930–937.

140 Mennitti LV et al: Type of fatty acids in maternal diets during pregnancy and/or lactation and metabolic consequences of the offspring. *J Nutr Biochem* 2015, 26:99–111.

141 Rudolph MC et al: Early infant adipose deposition is positively associated with the n-6 to n-3 fatty acid ratio in human milk independent of maternal BMI. *Int J Obes* 2017, 41:510–517.

142 Parra D et al: A diet rich in long chain omega-3 fatty acids modulates satiety in overweight and obese volunteers during weight loss. *Appetite* 2008, 51:676–680.

143 Wang L et al: A prospective study of erythrocyte polyunsaturated fatty acid, weight gain, and risk of becoming overweight or obese in middle-aged

and older women. *Eur J Nutr* 2015, www.ncbi.nlm.nih.gov/pmc /articles/PMC4587992; Thorsdottir I et al: Randomized trial of weight-loss-diets for young adults varying in fish and fish oil content. *Int J Obes* 2007, 31:1560–1566; Parra D et al: diet rich in long chain omega-3 fatty acids modulates satiety in overweight and obese volunteers during weight loss. *Appetite* 2008, 51:676–680; Cancer JD., Browning LM et al.: Additive benefits of long-chain n-3 polyunsaturated fatty acids and weight-loss in the management of cardiovascular disease risk in over-weight hyperinsulinaemic women. *Int J Obes* 2006, 30:1535–1544; Kunesova M et al.: The influence of n-3 polyunsaturated fatty acids and very low calorie diet during a short-term weight reducing regimen on weight loss and serum fatty acid composition in severely obese women. *Physiol Res* 2006, 55:63–72.

144 Simopoulos AP & DiNicolantonio JJ: The importance of a balanced ω-6 to ω-3 ratio in the prevention and management of obesity. *Open Heart* 2016, www.ncbi.nlm.nih.gov/pmc/articles/PMC5093368.

145 Knapton S: Obese three-year-old becomes youngest child diagnosed with Type 2 diabetes. *The Telegraph* 17.11.2015, www.telegraph.co.uk /news/health/news/11869249/Obese-three-year-old-becomes-youngest -child-di- agnosed-with-Type-2-diabetes.html.

146 CDC: A Report Card: Diabetes in the United States Infographic. May 15, 2024. https://www.cdc.gov/diabetes/communication-resources/diabetes -statistics.html.

147 American Diabetes Association: Statistics about Diabetes. Updated November 2023. https://diabetes.org/about-diabetes/statistics/about -diabetes; CDC National Center for Health Statistics: Death and Mortality. 2022. https://www.cdc.gov/nchs/fastats/deaths.htm.

148 Steven S et al: Very Low-Calorie Diet and 6 Months of Weight Stability in Type 2 Diabetes: Pathophysiological Changes in Responders and Nonresponders. *Diabetes Care* 2016, 39:808–815.

149 Albert BB et al: Higher omega-3 index is associated with increased insu-lin sensitivity and more favourable metabolic profile in middle-aged overweight men. *Sci Rep* 2014, www.ncbi.nlm.nih.gov/pmc/articles /PMC5381193.

150 Jacobo-Cejudo MG et al: Effect of n-3 Polyunsaturated Fatty Acid Supplementation on Metabolic and Inflammatory Biomarkers in Type

2 Diabetes Mellitus Patients. *Nutrients* 2017, www.ncbi.nlm.nih.gov /pmc/articles/PMC5490552.

151 DeRosa G et al: Effects of n-3 pufas on fasting plasma glucose and insulin resistance in patients with impaired fasting glucose or impaired glucose tolerance. *Biofactors* 2016, 42:316–322.

152 Sala-Vila A et al: Dietary Marine ω-3 Fatty Acids and Incident Sight-Threatening Retinopathy in Middle-Aged and Older Individuals With Type 2 Diabetes: Prospective Investigation From the PREDIMED Trial. *JAMA Ophthalmol* 2016, 134:1142–1149.

153 Rook GA: Hygiene hypothesis and autoimmune diseases. *Clin Rev Allergy Immunol* 2012, 42:5–15.

154 Okada H et al: The 'hygiene hypothesis' for autoimmune and allergic diseases: an update. *Clin Exp Immunol* 2010, 160:1–9.

155 Flint HJ et al: The impact of nutrition on intestinal bacterial communities. *Curr Opin Microbiol* 2017, 38:59–65.

156 Han M et al: Dietary Fiber Gap and Host Gut Microbiota. *Protein Pept Lett* 2017, 24:388–396.

157 Markle JG et al: Sex differences in the gut microbiome drive hormone-dependent regulation of autoimmunity. Science 2013, 339:1084–1088; Thion MS et al: Microbiome Influences Prenatal and Adult Microglia in a Sex-Specific Manner. *Cell* 2018, 172:500–516.

158 Costantini L et al: Impact of Omega-3 Fatty Acids on the Gut Microbiota. *Int J Mol Sci* 2017, www.ncbi.nlm.nih.gov/pmc/articles/PMC5751248.

159 Menni C et al: Omega-3 fatty acids correlate with gut microbiome diversity and production of N-carbamylglutamate in middle aged and elderly women. *Sci Rep* 2017, www.ncbi.nlm.nih.gov/pmc/articles /PMC5593975.

160 Niinistö S et al: Fatty acid status in infancy is associated with the risk of Type 1 diabetes-associated autoimmunity. *Diabetologia* 2017, 60:1223–1233.

161 Lamb M et al: The effect of childhood cow's milk intake and HLA-DR geneotype on risk of islet autoimmunity and Type 1 diabetes: The Diabetes Autoimmunity Study in the Young. *Pediatr Diabetes* 2015, 16: 31–33; Chia JSJ et al: A1 beta-casein milk protein and other environmental pre-disposing factors for Type 1 diabetes. *Nutr Diabetes* 2017, www.ncbi.nlm.nih.gov/pmc/articles/PMC5518798.

162 Fitzgerald KC et al: Diet quality is associated with disability and symptom severity in multiple sclerosis. *Neurology* 2018, 90:1–11.

163 Prietl B et al: Vitamin D and Immune Function. *Nutrients* 2013, 5: 2502–2521; Munger KL et al: 25-Hydroxyvitamin D deficiency and risk of MS among women in the Finnish Maternity Cohort. *Neurology* 2017 89:1578–1583.

164 Simopoulos AP: Omega-3 fatty acids in inflammation and autoimmune diseases. *J Am Coll Nutr* 2002, 21:495–505.

165 Rajaei E et al: The Effect of Omega-3 Fatty Acids in Patients With Active Rheumatoid Arthritis Receiving DMARDs Therapy: Double-Blind Randomized Controlled Trial. *Glob J Health Sci* 2016, 8: 18–25.

166 Thomsen SF: Epidemiology and natural history of atopic diseases. *Eur Clin Respir J* 2015, www.ncbi.nlm.nih.gov/pmc/articles/PMC4629767.

167 Furuhjelm C et al: Allergic disease in infants up to 2 years of age in relation to plasma omega-3 fatty acids and maternal fish oil supplementation in pregnancy and lactation. *Pediatr Allergy Immunol* 2011, 22:505–514; Bisgaard H et al: Fish Oil-Derived Fatty Acids in Pregnancy and Wheeze and Asthma in Offspring. *N Engl J Med* 2016, 375:2530–2539.

168 Warstedt K et al: High levels of omega-3 fatty acids in milk from omega-3 fatty acid-supplemented mothers are related to less immunoglobulin E-associated disease in infancy. *Acta Paediatr* 2016, 105:1337–1347.

169 Bhanegaonkar A et al: Economic Burden of Atopic Dermatitis in High-Risk Infants Receiving Cow's Milk or Partially Hydrolyzed 100% Whey-Based Formula. *J Pediatr* 2015, 166:1145–1151.

170 D'Vaz N et al: Fish oil supplementation in early infancy modulates developing infant immune responses. *Clin Exp Allergy* 2012, 42:1206–1216.

171 Hansen S et al: Fish oil supplementation during pregnancy and allergic respiratory disease in the adult offspring. *J Allergy Clin Immunol* 2017, 139:104–111.

172 Smolokoff A: American diets falling short in Omega-3 fatty acids. *SupplySide Food & Beverage Journal.* May 26, 2021.https://www.supplysidefbj.com /fat-oils/american-diets-falling-short-in-omega-3-fatty-acids.

173 Serhan CN et al: The resolution code of acute inflammation: Novel pro-resolving lipid mediators in resolution. *Semin Immunol* 2015, 27:200–215; Calder PC: Marine omega-3 fatty acids and inflammatory processes: effects, mechanisms and clinical relevance. *Biochim Biophys Acta* 2015;1851:469–484; Kunisawa J et al: Dietary ω3 fatty acid exerts anti-allergic effect through the conversion to 17,18-epoxyeicosatetraenoic

acid in the gut. *Sci Rep* 2015, www.ncbi.nlm.nih.gov/pmc/articles /PMC446425.

174 Ramsden CE: Breathing Easier with Fish Oil - A New Approach to Preventing Asthma? *N Engl J Med* 2016, 375:2596–2598.

175 Maroon JC & Bost JW: Omega-3 fatty acids (fish oil) as an anti-inflammatory: an alternative to nonsteroidal anti-inflammatory drugs for discogenic pain. *Surg Neurol* 2006, 65:326–331.

176 Cancer. WHO February 2018, www.who.int/mediacentre/factsheets /fs297/en/.

177 Jing K et al: Omega-3 polyunsaturated fatty acids and cancer. *Anticancer Agents Med Chem* 2013, 13:1162–1177.

178 Hunter P: The inflammation theory of disease. The growing realization that chronic inflammation is crucial in many diseases opens new avenues for treatment. *EMBO Rep* 2012, 13: 968–970.

179 Patterson WL 3rd & Georgel PT: Breaking the cycle: the role of omega-3 polyunsaturated fatty acids in inflammation-driven cancers. *Biochem Cell Biol* 2014, 92:321–328; Zhang Q et al: Resolution of Cancer-Promoting Inflammation: A New Approach for Anticancer Therapy. *Front Immunol* 2017, www.ncbi.nlm.nih.gov/pmc/articles/PMC5288347.

180 Huerta-Yépez S et al: Role of diets rich in omega-3 and omega-6 in the development of cancer. *Bol Med Hosp Infant Mex* 2016, 73:446–456.

181 Rather IA et al: The Sources of Chemical Contaminants in Food and Their Health Implications. *Front Pharmacol* 2017, www.ncbi.nlm.nih .gov/pmc/articles/PMC5699236.

182 Ghorbanihaghjo A et al: Protective effect of fish oil supplementation on DNA damage induced by cigarette smoking. *J Health Popul Nutr* 201, 31:343–349.

183 Gallagher RP et al: Plasma levels of polychlorinated biphenyls and risk of cutaneous malignant melanoma: a preliminary study. *Int J Cancer* 2011, 128:1872–1880.

184 Donat-Vargas C et al: Dietary polychlorinated biphenyls, long-chain n-3 poly- unsaturated fatty acids and incidence of malignant melanoma. *Eur J Cancer* 2017, 72:137–143.

185 Bishop KS et al: An investigation into the association between DNA damage and dietary fatty acid in men with prostate cancer. *Nutrients* 2015, 7:405–422.

186 Torfadottir JE et al: Milk intake in early life and risk of advanced prostate cancer. *Am J Epidemiol* 2012, 175:144–153; Bouvard V et al: Carcinogenicity of consumption of red and processed meat. *Lancet Oncol* 2015, 16:1599–1600.

187 Bernstein C et al: Chapter 16: DNA Damage, DNA Repair and Cancer. *New Research Directions in DNA Repair*. Intech Open, May 22, 2013. www.intechopen.com/books/new-research-directions-in-dna-repair /dna-dam- age-dna-repair-and-cancer.

188 Monzavi-Karbassi B et al: Tumor-Associated Glycans and Immune Surveillance. *Vaccines* 2013, 1:174–203.

189 Liang P et al: Effect of Dietary Omega-3 Fatty Acids on Tumor-Associated Macrophages and Prostate Cancer Progression. *Prostate* 2016, 76:1293–1302; Pahl J & Cerwenka A: Tricking the balance: NK cells in anti-cancer immunity. *Immunobiology* 2017, 222:11–20.

190 Newell M et al: A Critical Review on the Effect of Docosahexaenoic Acid (DHA) on Cancer Cell Cycle Progression. *Int J Mol Sci* 2017, www.ncbi.nlm. nih.gov/pmc/articles/PMC5578173.

191 Abdi J et al: Omega-3 fatty acids, EPA and DHA induce apoptosis and enhance drug sensitivity in multiple myeloma cells but not in normal peripheral mononuclear cells. *J Nutr Biochem* 2014, 25:1254–1262.

192 Song EA & Kim H: Docosahexaenoic Acid Induces Oxidative DNA Damage and Apoptosis, and Enhances the Chemosensitivity of Cancer Cells. *Int J Mol Sci* 2016, www.ncbi.nlm.nih.gov/pmc/articles /PMC5000655.

193 Jing K et al: Omega-3 polyunsaturated fatty acids and cancer. *Anticancer Agents Med Chem* 2013, 13:1162–1177.

194 Kang JX & Liu A: The role of the tissue omega-6/omega-3 fatty acid ratio in regulating tumor angiogenesis. *Cancer Metastasis Rev* 2013, 32:201–210.

195 Zanoaga O et al: Implications of dietary ω-3 and ω-6 polyunsaturated fatty acids in breast cancer. *Exp Ther Med* 2018, 15:1167–1176.

196 Yang B at el: Ratio of n-3/n-6 PUFAs and risk of breast cancer: a meta-analysis of 274135 adult females from 11 independent prospective studies. *BMC Cancer* 2014, www.ncbi.nlm.nih.gov/pmc/articles/PMC4016587.

197 Ibid.

198 Lavado-García J et al: Long-chain omega-3 polyunsaturated fatty acid dietary intake is positively associated with bone mineral density in normal and osteopenic Spanish women. *PLoS One* 2018, www.ncbi.nlm .nih.gov/pmc/articles/PMC5755813.

199 Kelly OJ et al: Long-chain polyunsaturated fatty acids may mutually benefit both obesity and osteoporosis. *Nutr Res* 2013, 33:521–533.

200 Reginster JY & Burlet N: Osteoporosis: a still increasing prevalence. *Bone* 2006, 38:4–9.

201 Leboime A et al: Osteoporosis and mortality. *Joint Bone Spine* 2010, 77:107–112.

202 Tachtsis B et al: Potenzial Roles of n-3 PUFAs during Skeletal Muscle Growth and Regeneration. *Nutrients* 2018, www.ncbi.nlm.nih.gov/pmc /articles/PMC5872727.

203 Lalia AZ et al: Influence of omega-3 fatty acids on skeletal muscle protein metabolism and mitochondrial bioenergetics in older adults. *Aging* 2017, 9:1096–1129.

204 Jouris KB et al: The Effect of Omega-3 Fatty Acid Supplementation on the Inflammatory Response to eccentric strength exercise. *J Sports Sci Med* 2011, 10:432–438.

PART IV: A THREAT TO GLOBAL HEALTH

1 Grantham-McGregor S et al: Developmental potential in the first 5 years for children in developing countries. *Lancet* 2007, 369:60–70.

2 WHO: Micronutrient deficiency (accessed 1/24/18), www.who.int /nutrition/topics/vad/en/.

3 FAO: Global Trends and Future Challenges for the Work of the Organization. In: 69th Session of the Committee on Commodity Problems 2012, http://fao. org/docrep/meeting/025/md883E.pdf.

4 Mashavave G et al: Dried blood spot omega-3 and omega-6 long chain poly-unsaturated fatty acid levels in 7–9 year old Zimbabwean children: a cross sectional study. *BMC Clin Pathol* 2016, www.ncbi.nlm.nih.gov /pmc/articles/PMC4974798.

5 Barbarich BN et al: Polyunsaturated fatty acids and anthropometric indices of children in rural China. *Eur J Clin Nutr* 2006, 60:1100–1107; Yakes EA et al: Intakes and breast-milk concentrations of essential fatty acids are low among Bangladeshi women with 24–48-month-old children. *BR J Nutr* 2011, 105:1660–1670.

6 Michaelsen KF et al: Food sources and intake of n-6 and n-3 fatty acids in low-income countries with emphasis on infants, young children (6–24 months), and pregnant and lactating women. *Mater. Child Nutr* 2011, 7:124–140.

7 Cordain L et al: Origins and evolution of the Western diet: health implications for the 21st century. *Am J Clin Nutr* 2005, 81:341–354.

8 Conzade R et al: Prevalence and Predictors of Subclinical Micronutrient Deficiency in German Older Adults: Results from the Population-Based KORA-Age Study. *Nutrients* 2017, www.ncbi.nlm.nih.gov/pmc/articles /PMC5748727.

9 Rabenberg M et al: Vitamin D status among adults in Germany—results from the German Health Interview and Examination Survey for Adults (DEGS1.) *BMC Public Health* 2015, www.ncbi.nlm.nih.gov /pmc/articles/PMC4499202.

10 National Institutes of Health: Vitamin D Fact Sheet for Professionals. Updated July 26, 2024. https://ods.od.nih.gov/factsheets/VitaminD -HealthProfessional/.

11 Nehls M: *Alzheimer ist heilbar—Rechtzeitig zurück in ein gesundes Leben.* Heyne 2017, 224–225.

12 Bewegung und Omega-3-Fette helfen Hirn kaum. *Ärzte Zeitung* online 31.08.2015, www.aerztezeitung.de/medizin/krankheiten/demenz/arti- cle /892873/demenz-bewegung-omega-3-fette-helfen-hirn-kaum.html.

13 Sydenham et al: Omega 3 fatty acid for the prevention of cognitive decline and dementia. *Cochrane Database Syst Rev* 2012, www.ncbi.nlm .nih.gov/pubmed/22696350.

14 Tao L: Oxidation of Polyunsaturated Fatty Acids and its Impact on Food Quality and Human Health. *Advances in Food Technology and Nutritional Sciences* 2015, https://openventio.org/Volume1-Issue6/Oxidation-of-Poly -unsaturated-Fatty-Acids-and-its-Impact-on-Food-Quality-and-Human -Health-AFTNSOJ-1–123.pdf.

15 Albert BB et al: Fish oil supplements in New Zealand are highly oxi-dised and do not meet label content of n-3 PUFA. *Sci Rep* 2015, www.ncbi.nlm.nih.gov/pmc/articles/PMC4300506; Albert T et al: Omega-3 fish oil products and responding to a flawed research study. 2015, www .nutraingredients-usa.com/Research/Omega-3-fish-oil-products -and-responding-to-a-flawed-research-study.

16 Kitson AP et al: Pan-frying salmon in an eicosapentaenoic acid (EPA) and docosahexaenoic acid (DHA) enriched margarine prevents EPA and DHA loss. *Food Chemistry* 2009, 114: 927–932.

17 Halvorsen BL & Blomhoff R: Determination of lipid oxidation products in vegetable oils and marine omega-3 supplements. *Food Nutr Res* 2011, www. ncbi.nlm.nih.gov/pmc/articles/PMC3118035.

18 Patterson AC et al: The percentage of DHA in erythrocytes can detect non-adherence to advice to increase EPA and DHA intakes. *Br J Nutr* 2014, 111:270–278.

19 Eckert N: Omega-3-Fettsäuren schützen laut Metaanalyse doch nicht das Herz von Hochrisikopatienten—Experten sind skeptisch. 2018, https://deutsch.medscape.com/artikelansicht/4906739.

20 Modified from Radcliffe JE et al: Controversies in omega-3 efficacy and novel concepts for application. *J Nutr & Intermediary Metab* 2016, www. sciencedirect.com/science/article/pii/S2352385916300020.

21 Superko HR et al: Omega-3 fatty acid blood levels: clinical significance and controversy. *Circulation* 2013, 128:2154–2161.

22 Ameur A et al: Genetic adaptation of fatty-acid metabolism: a human-specific haplotype increasing the biosynthesis of long-chain omega-3 and omega-6 fatty acids. *On J Hum Genet* 2012, 90:809–820.

23 Block RC et al: Determinants of blood cell omega-3 fatty acid content. *Open Biomark J* 2008, 1:1–6.

24 Rizos EC et al: Association between omega-3 fatty acid supplementation and risk of major cardiovascular disease events: a systematic review and me-ta-analysis. *JAMA* 2012, 308:1024–1033.

25 Itakura H et al: Relationships between plasma fatty acid composition and coronary artery disease. *J Atheroscler Thromb* 2011, 18:99–107.

26 EFSA Panel on Dietetic Products, Nutrition and Allergies (NDA); Scientific Opinion on the substantiation of health claims related to EPA, DHA, DPA and maintenance of normal blood pressure (ID 502), maintenance of normal HDL-cholesterol concentrations (ID 515), maintenance of normal (fasting) blood concentrations of triglycerides (ID 517), maintenance of normal LDL-cholesterol concentrations (ID 528, 698) and maintenance of joints (ID 503, 505, 507, 511, 518, 524, 526, 535, 537) pursuant to Article 13(1) of Regulation (EC) No 1924/2006 on request from the European Commission. *EFSA Journal* 2009, www .efsa.europa.eu/de/efsajournal/pub/1263.

27 Koletzko B et al: The roles of long-chain polyunsaturated fatty acids in pregnancy, lactation and infancy: Review of current knowledge and consensus recommendations. *J Perinat Med* 2008, 36:5–14; European Food Safety Authority Scientific opinion on dietary reference values for fats, including saturated fatty acids, polyunsaturated fatty acids, mono-unsaturated fatty acids, trans fatty acids, and cholesterol. *EFSA J* 2010, http://onlinelibrary. wiley.com/doi/10.2903/j.efsa.2010.1461/epdf.

28 Dietary Guidelines for Americans. Washington, DC: U.S. Government Printing Office 2010, https://health.gov/dietaryguidelines/dga2010/dietaryguide- lines2010.pdf.

29 EFSA Panel on Dietetic Products, Nutrition and Allergies (NDA): Scientific Opinion on the Tolerable Upper Intake Level of eicosapen-taenoic acid (EPA), docosahexaenoic acid (DHA) and docosapentaenoic acid (DPA). *EFSA Journal* Vol. 10, Issue 7 July 2012. http://onlinelib rary.wiley.com/doi/10.2903/j.efsa.2012.2815/epdf.

30 Coletta JM et al: Omega-3 Fatty acids and pregnancy. *Rev Obstet Gynecol* 2010, 3:163–171; US Food and Drug Administration Web site, 2010, What you need to know about mercury in fish and shellfish. www.fda.gov/food/foodsafety/product-specificinformation/seafood/food bornepathogenscontaminants/methylmercury/ucm115662.htm.

31 Frithsen I & Goodnight W: Awareness and implications of fish con-sumption advisories in a women's health setting. *J Reprod Med* 2009, 54:267–272; Bloomingdale A et al: A qualitative study of fish consump-tion during pregnancy. *Am J Clin Nutr* 2010, 92:1234–1240; Coletta JM et al: Omega-3 Fatty acids and pregnancy. *Rev Obstet Gynecol* 2010, 3:163–171.

32 American Heart Association: Fish and Omega-3 Fatty Acids. www.heart.org/HEARTORG/HealthyLiving/HealthyEating/HealthyDiet-Goals/Fish-and-Omega-3-Fatty-Acids_UCM_303248_Article.jsp#. Wmb8KvlS-1KI.

33 Flock MR et al: Long-chain omega-3 fatty acids: Time to establish a dietary reference intake. *Nutr Rev* 2013, 71:692–707.

34 Patterson AC et al: Omega-3 polyunsaturated fatty acid blood biomark-ers increase linearly in men and women after tightly controlled intakes of 0.25, 0.5, and 1 g/d of EPA + DHA. *Nutr Res* 2015, 35:1040–1051.

35 Côté S et al: Very high concentrations of n-3 fatty acids in peri- and post-menopausal Inuit women from Greenland. *Int J Circumpolar Health* 2004, 63:298–301.

36 Eckert N: Omega-3-Fettsäuren schützen laut Metaanalyse doch nicht das Herz von Hochrisikopatienten—Experten sind skeptisch. 2018, https://deutsch.medscape.com/artikelansicht/4906739.

37 Thuppal SV et al: Discrepancy between Knowledge and Perceptions of Dietary Omega-3 Fatty Acid Intake Compared with the Omega-3 Index. *Nutrients* 2017, www.ncbi.nlm.nih.gov/pmc/articles/PMC5622690.

38 Modified from Stark KD et al: Global survey of the omega-3 fatty acids, docosahexaenoic acid and eicosapentaenoic acid in the blood stream of healthy adults. *Prog Lipid Res,* 2016, 63:132–152.

39 Modified from Food and Agriculture Organization of the United Nations (FAO): The state of world fisheries and aquaculture 2016, www.fao.org/3/a- i5555e.pdf, Page 77.

40 Pauly D & Zeller D: Catch reconstructions reveal that global marine fisheries catches are higher than reported and declining. *Nat Commun* 2016, www. ncbi.nlm.nih.gov/pmc/articles/PMC4735634/pdf.

41 Mohanty BP et al: DHA and EPA Content and Fatty Acid Profile of 39 Food Fishes from India. *Biomed Res Int* 2016;2016, www.ncbi.nlm.nih.gov/pmc/articles/PMC4989070.

42 Sprague M et al: Impact of sustainable feeds on omega-3 long-chain fatty acid levels in farmed Atlantic salmon, 2006–2015. *Scientific Reports* 2016, www.nature.com/articles/srep21892; www.heartfoundation.org.au/imag- es/uploads/main/Programs/Sources_of_omega_3.pdf.

43 Salem Jr N & Eggersdorfer M: Is the world supply of omega-3 fatty acids adequate for optimal human nutrition? *Curr Opin Clin Nutr Metab Care* 2015, 18:147–154.

44 United Nations: World population projected to reach 9.8 billion in 2050, and 11.2 billion in 2100. 21.06.2017, www.un.org/development/desa/en/news/population/world-population-prospects-2017.html.

45 United Nations Convention on the Law of the Sea .1982, www.admin.ch/opc/de/official-compilation/2009/3209.pdf.

46 Die Zukunft der Fische—die Fischerei der Zukunft. World Ocean Review: Mit den Meeren leben. 2013, http://worldoceanreview.com/wp-content/downloads/wor2/WOR2_gesamt.pdf

47   FAO: General situation of world fish stocks. 2010, http://fao.org/newsroom/
     common/ecg/1000505/en/stocks.pdf.

48   Bale R: One of the World's Biggest Fisheries Is on the Verge of
     Collapse. National Geographic Wildlife Watch 29.08. 2016, https://news.
     nationalgeographic.com/2016/08/wildlife-south-china-sea-overfishing
     -threatens-collapse/.

49   Worm B et al: Impacts of biodiversity loss on ocean ecosystem services.
     Science 2006, 314:787–790.

50   Aquakultur—Proteinlieferant für die Welt. *World Ocean Review* 2013,
     http://worldoceanreview.com/wor-2/aquakultur/proteinliefer-ant-fuer
     -die-welt/.

51   Sargent JR et al: The metabolism of phospholipids and polyunsaturated
     fatty acids in fish. Aquaculture: Fundamental and Applied Research.
     Coastal and Estuarine Studies 1993, 43:103–124.

52   Sprague M et al: Impact of sustainable feeds on omega-3 long-chain
     fatty acid levels in farmed Atlantic salmon, 2006–2015. *Sci Rep* 2016,
     www.ncbi. nlm.nih.gov/pubmed/26899924.

53   Mozaffarian D & Rimm EB: Fish intake, contaminants and human
     health-evaluating the risks and the benefits. *JAMA* 2006, 296:1885–189.

54   Hackshaw A et al: Low cigarette consumption and risk of coronary
     heart disease and stroke: meta-analysis of 141 cohort studies in 55 study
     reports. *BMJ* 2018, https://doi.org/10.1136/bmj.j5855.

55   Topiwala A, Allan C L, Valkanova V, Zsoldos E, Filippini N, Sexton C et al.:
     Moderate alcohol consumption as risk factor for adverse brain outcomes
     and cognitive decline: longitudinal cohort study BMJ 2017; 357:j2353
     doi:10.1136/bmj.j2353, https://www.bmj.com/content/357/bmj.j2353.

56   Chasek, Pamela: Stockholm Convention on Persistent Organic Pollutants.
     Earth Negotiations Bulletin, 2023, https://enb.iisd.org/articles/Stockholm
     -convention.

57   Schneutz R: Milliarden Tonnen an biologisch nicht abbaubaren Plastikmüll
     haben sich in der Umwelt angesammelt. *Telepolis* 2017, www.heise.de
     /forum/Telepolis/Kommentare/Milliarden-Tonnen-an-biologisch-nicht
     -abbau-baren-Plastikmuell-haben-sich-in-der-Umwelt-angesammelt
     /Weichmacher-PCB-das-dreckige-Dutzend-verbotener-Chemikalien
     /posting-30740056/show/.

58   Seynsche M: PCB hat katastrophale Folgen für Meeressäuger. *Deutsch
     landfunk* 2016, www.deutschlandfunk.de/schwertwale-pcb-hat-katastrophale-
     folgen-fuer-meeressaeuger.676.de.html?dram%3Aarticle_id=357572.

59 Meeker JD & Hauser R: Exposure to polychlorinated biphenyls (PCBs) and male reproduction. *Syst Biol Reprod Med* 2010, 56:122–131.

60 Cohn BA et al: Polychlorinated biphenyl (PCB) exposure in mothers and time to pregnancy in daughters. *Reprod Toxicol* 2011, 31:290–296.

61 Pocar P et al: Effects of polychlorinated biphenyls in CD-1 mice: reproductive toxicity and intergenerational transmission. *Toxicological Sciences* 2012, 126:213–226.

62 https://www.researchgate.net/blog/another-ocean-garbage-patch.

63 World Economic Forum: The New Plastics Economy Rethinking the future of plastics. 2017, www3.weforum.org/docs/WEF_The_New _Plastics_Economy.pdf.

64 Rochman CM et al: Polybrominated diphenyl ethers (PBDEs) in fish tissue may be an indicator of plastic contamination in marine habitats. *Sci Total Environ* 2014, 476–477:622–633.

65 Savoca MS et al: Odours from marine plastic debris induce food search behaviours in a forage fish. *Proc Biol Sci* 2017, www.ncbi.nlm.nih.gov /pmc/articles/PMC5563810.

66 Coates, Ashley: Ocean plastic cleanup: A 23-year-old's mission to take rubbish out of our seas. Independent, 2017, https://www.independent.co .uk/climate-change/news/ocean-plastic-cleanup-rubbish-seas-take-out -23-year-old-boyan-slat-north-sea-pacific-microplastics-great-pacific -garbage-patch-a7880321.html.

67 do Costa S et al: Endocrine interruption instigated by triorganotin (IV) mixes: Impacts in the regenerative and hereditary capacity. *Int J Genetics and Genomics* 2014, 1:1–9.

68 Heblik D: Ist Fisch noch genießbar? *UGB Forum*, www.ugb.de/lebensmit-tel-im-test/ist-fisch-noch-geniessbar/druckansicht.pdf.

69 Repossi A et al: Bisphenol A in Edible Part of Seafood. *Ital J Food Saf* 2016, www.ncbi.nlm.nih.gov/pmc/articles/PMC5076740; Cabado AG et al: Migration of BADGE (bisphenol A diglycidyl-ether) and BFDGE (bisphenol F diglycidyl-ether) in canned seafood. *Food Chem Toxicol* 2008, 46:1674–1680.

70 Acconcia F et al: Molecular Mechanisms of Action of BPA. *Dose Response* 2015, www.ncbi.nlm.nih.gov/pmc/articles/PMC4679188.

71 Rahman MS et al: Bisphenol-A Affects Male Fertility via Fertility-related Proteins in Spermatozoa. *SCI Rep* 2015, www.ncbi.nlm.nih.gov/pmc /articles/PMC4360475.

72 Zheng H et al: Genome-wide alteration in DNA hydroxymethylation in the sperm from bisphenol A-exposed men. *PLoS* One 2017, www.ncbi .nlm.nih. Gov/pmc/articles/PMC5459435.

73 Focardi S et al: PCB congeners, DDTs and hexachlorobenzene in Antarctic fish from Terra Nova Bay (Ross Sea.) *Antarctic Science* 1992, 4:151–154.

74 Nash B et al: A nutritional-toxicological assessment of Antarctic krill oil versus fish oil dietary supplements. *Nutrients* 2014, 6:3382–3402.

75 Atkinson A et al: A re-appraisal of the total biomass and annual production of Antarctic krill. *Deep-Sea Research I* 2009, 56:727–740.

76 Nicol S et al: The fishery for Antarctic krill—recent developments. *Fish and Fisheries* 2012, 13:30–40.

77 Nicol, S., Foster, J. and Kawaguchi, S.: The fishery for Antarctic krill—recent developments. Fish and Fisheries, 13: 30-40. 2012, https://onlinelibrary.wiley.com/doi/10.1111/j.1467-2979.2011.00406.x.

78 Moranmarch S: Team Tracks a Food Supply at the End of the World. *New York Times* 2012, www.nytimes.com/2012/03/13/science/tracking -antarc- tic-krill-as-more-is-harvested-for-omega-3-pills.html.

79 Hill SL et al: Modelling Southern Ocean ecosystems: krill, the food-web, and the impacts of harvesting. *Biol Rev Camb Philos Soc* 2006, 81:581–608.

80 Boyce DG et al: Global phytoplankton decline over the past century. *Nature* 2010, 466:591–596.

81 Cool Antarctica: Antarctica and Climate Change the Effects on Antarctica. www.coolantarctica.com/Antarctica%20fact%20file/science/global _warming.php.

82 Trivelpiece WZ et al: Variability in krill biomass links harvesting and climate warming to penguin population changes in Antarctica. *Proc Natl Acad Sci* USA. 2011, 108:7625–7628.

PART V: OVERCOMING THE GLOBAL CRISIS WITH MICROALGAE OIL

1 Wells ML et al: Algae as nutritional and functional food sources: revisiting our understanding. *J Appl Phycol* 2017, 29:949–982.

2 Guiry MD: How many species of algae are there? *J Phycol* 2012, 48:1057–1063.

3   Cardozo KH et al: Metabolites from algae with economical impact. *Comp Biochem Physiol C Toxicol Pharmacol* 2007, 146:60–78.

4   Abdo SM: Potencial Production of Omega Fatty Acids from Microalgae. *Int J Pharm Sci Rev* 2015, 35:210–215; Hu H et al: Isolation and Characterization of a Mesophilic Arthrospira maxima Strain Capable of Producing Docosahexaenoic Acid. *J Microbiol Biotechnol* 2011, 21:697–702.

5   Shapiro JA: Living Organisms Author Their Read-Write Genomes in Evolution. *Biology* 2017, www.ncbi.nlm.nih.gov/pmc/articles/PMC5745 447.

6   McFadden GI: Origin and evolution of plastids and photosynthesis in eukaryotes. *Cold Spring Harb Perspect Biol* 2014, www.ncbi.nlm.nih .gov/pmc/articles/PMC3970417.

7   Belasco W: Algae Burgers for a Hungry World? The Rise and Fall of Chlorella Cuisine. *Technology and Culture* 1997, 3: 608–634.

8   Subramoniam A et al: Chlorophyll revisited: anti-inflammatory activities of chlorophyll a and inhibition of expression of TNF-α gene by the same. *Inflammation* 2012, 35:959–966.

9   Becker EW: Micro-algae as a source of protein. *Biotechnol Adv* 2007, 25:207–210.

10 Vazhappilly R & Chen F: Eicosapentaenoic Acid and Docosahexaenoic Acid Production Potenzial of Microalgae and Their Heterotrophic Growth. *JAOCS* 1998, 75:393–397; Yongmanitchai W & Ward OP: Screening of algae for potential alternative sources of eicosapentaenoic acid. *Phytochemistry* 1991, 9:2963–2967.

11 Sharma K & Schenk PM: Rapid induction of omega-3 fatty acids (EPA) in Nannochloropsis sp. by UV-C radiation. *Biotechnol Bioeng* 2015, 112:1243–1249.

12 Tessari P et al: Essential amino acids: master regulators of nutrition and environmental footprint? *SCI Rep* 2016, www.ncbi.nlm.nih.gov/pmc /articles/PMC4897092.

13 Moomaw W et al: Cutting Out the Middle Fish: Marine Microalgae as the Next Sustainable Omega-3 Fatty Acids and Protein Source. *Industrial Biotechnology* 2017, 13:234–243.

14 Ren LJ et al: Development of a stepwise aeration control strategy for efficient docosahexaenoic acid production by Schizochytrium sp. *Appl Microbiol Biotechnol* 2010, 87:1649–1656.

15 DSM Nutritional Products, propiertärer Stamm: Kyle DJ: 20—Future Development of Single Cell Oils. *Single Cell Oils* 2010, 2:439–451.

16 Raghu-Kumar S: Schizochytrium mangrovei sp. nov., a thraustochytrid from mangroves in India. *Transact Bri Myc Soc* 1988, 90:627–631.

17 Leyland B et al: Are Thraustochytrids algae? *Fungal Biol* 2017, 121: 835–840.

18 Durchführungsbeschluss der Kommission vom 14.Juli 2014 zur Genehmigung des Inverkehrbringens von Öl aus der Mikroalge Schizochytrium sp. als neuartige Lebensmittelzutat im Sinne der Verordnung (EG) Nr. 258/97 des Europäischen Parlaments und des Rates und zur Aufhebung der Entscheidungen 2003/427/EG und 2009 /778/EG. http://eur-lex.europa.eu/le-gal-content/DE/TXT/PDF/?uri =CELEX:32014D0463&from=DE.

19 Barclay WR et al: Heterotropic production of long chain omega-3-fatty acids utilizing algae and algae-like microorganism. *J Appl Phycol* 1994; 6:123–129.

20 Zhang Y et al: Effect of malate on docosahexaenoic acid production from Schizochytrium sp. B4D1. *Electronic Journal of Biotechnology* 2016, 19: 56–60.

21 World Population Review: Sugar Consumption by Country 2024. https://worldpopulationreview.com/country-rankings/sugar-consumption -by-country.

22 Adarme-Vega TC et al: Microalgal biofactories: a promising approach towards sustainable omega-3 fatty acid production. *Microb Cell Fact* 2012, www.ncbi.nlm.nih.gov/pmc/articles/PMC3465194.

23 Fraunhofer Institut für Grenzflächen- und Bioverfahrenstechnik: Algen—Nachhaltige Rohstoffquelle für Wertstoffe und Energie. www .igb.fraunhofer.de/content/dam/igb/de/documents/broschueren/ubt /1506_BR-ubt_al- gen_de.pdf.

24 Bergmann P et al: Suspension Culture of Microorganisms (Algae and Cyanobacteria) Under Phototrophic Conditions. Industrial Scale Suspension Culture of Living Cells. *Wiley-VCH* 2014, 6:199–222.

25 Medipally SR et al: Microalgae as sustainable renewable energy feed-stock for biofuel production. *Biomed Res Int* 2015, www.ncbi.nlm.nih .gov/pmc/articles/PMC4385614.

26 Wright CK & Wimberly MC: Recent land use change in the Western Corn Belt threatens grasslands and wetlands. *Proc Natl Acad Sci* USA 2013, 110:4134–4139.

27 Carstens P: Erneuerbare Energien Biogas aus der Algenfabrik. (Page visited 02/2018), www.geo.de/natur/nachhaltigkeit/3806-rtkl-erneuerbare -ener- gien-biogas-aus-der-algenfabrik.

28 Schrader C: Wie steht es um die Einlagerung von Kohlendioxid? *Spektrum*.de 14.3.2018, www.spektrum.de/news/wie-steht-es-um-die -einlagerung-von- kohlendioxid/1549421.

29 Glaser B: Prehistorically modified soils of central Amazonia: a model for sustainable agriculture in the twenty-first century. *Biological Sciences* 2007, 362:187–196.

30 Scheub U & Stefan Schwarzer S: *Die Humusrevolution: Wie wir den Boden heilen, das Klima retten und die Ernährungswende schaffen.* oekom 2017.

31 Wen Z & Johnson MB: Microalgae as a Feedstock for Biofuel Production. *Virginia Cooperative Extension* 2009, http://pubs.ext.vt.edu/content/dam /pubs_ext_vt_edu/422/442–886/442–886_pdf.pdf.

32 ibid..

33 Ryckebosch E et al: Stability of omega-3 LC-PUFA-rich photoautotrophic microalgal oils compared to commercially available omega-3 LC-PUFA oils. *J Agric Food Chem* 2013, 61:10145–10155.

34 Ryckebosch E et al: Nutritional evaluation of microalgae oils rich in omega-3 long chain polyunsaturated fatty acids as an alternative for fish oil. *Food Chem* 2014, 160:393–400.

35 Kagan ML et al: Acute appearance of fatty acids in human plasma— a comparative study between polar-lipid rich oil from the microalgae Nannochloropsis oculata and krill oil in healthy young males. *Lipids Health Dis* 2013, www.ncbi.nlm.nih.gov/pmc/articles/PMC3718725.

36 Ulven SM & Holven KB: Comparison of bioavailability of krill oil versus fish oil and health effect. *Vasc Health Risk Manag* 2015, 11:511–524.

37 Lang I et al: Fatty acid profiles and their distribution patterns in microalgae: a comprehensive analysis of more than 2000 strains from the SAG culture collection. *BMC Plant Biol* 2011, www.ncbi.nlm.nih.gov/pmc /articles/PMC3175173.

38 Steinrücken P et al: Bioprospecting North Atlantic microalgae with fast growth and high polyunsaturated fatty acid (PUFA) content for microalgae-based technologies. *Algal Res* 2017, www.ncbi.nlm.nih.gov /pmc/arti- cles/PMC5614095.

39 Lane J: Big Algae chases Omega-3 dominance: DSM, Evonik underway on $200M algae project in Nebraska. *Biofuels Digest* 2018, www.bio fuelsdigest.com/bdigest/2018/02/15/big-algae-chases-omega-3-dominance -dsm- evonik-underway-on-200m-algae-project-in-nebraska.

40 Fan J et al: Genomic Foundation of Starch-to-Lipid Switch in Oleaginous Chlorella spp. *Plant Physiol* 2015, 169:2444–2461.

41 Amjad Khan W et al: Bioengineered Plants Can Be a Useful Source of Omega-3 Fatty Acids. *Biomed Res Int* 2017, www.ncbi.nlm.nih.gov /pmc/articles/PMC5339522.

42 Sprague M et al: Microbial and genetically engineered oils as replacements for fish oil in aquaculture feeds. *Biotechnol Lett* 2017, 39:1599–1609.

43 Coxworth B: Scientists take the fish out of fish food. *New Atlas* 2016, https://newatlas.com/microalgae-fish-oil/43707; Sarker PK et al: Towards Sustainable Aquafeeds: Complete Substitution of Fish Oil with Marine Microalga Schizochytrium sp. Improves Growth and Fatty Acid Deposition in Juvenile Nile Tilapia (Oreochromis niloticus). *PLoS One* 2016, www.ncbi. nlm.nih.gov/pmc/articles/PMC4892564.

44 DSM and Evonik establish Veramaris joint venture. 2018, http: //corporate.evonik.com/en/media/press_releases/Pages/news-details.aspx ?news-id=72670.

45 DGE: The German Nutrition Society. www.dge.de/wissenschaft/referenz werte/jod.

46 Lefton, Jennifer: Benefits of Copper and How to Get Enough. Verywell Health 2024, https://www.verywellhealth.com/copper-benefits-4178854.

47 Marshall TM: Lithium as a nutrient. *J Am Phys Surg* 2015, 20: 104–109, www.jpands.org/vol20no4/marshall.pdf.

48 Selenium. Harvard T.H. Chan School of Public Health, 2023, https: //nutritionsource.hsph.harvard.edu/selenium/.

49 Vitamin A and Carotenoids. National Institutes of Health, 2023, https://ods.od.nih.gov/factsheets/VitaminA-HealthProfessional/.

50 Thiamin. National Institutes of Health, 2023, https://ods.od.nih.gov /factsheets/Thiamin-HealthProfessional/.

51 Institute of Medicine (US) Standing Committee on the Scientific
    Evaluation of Dietary Reference Intakes and its Panel on Folate, Other
    B Vitamins, and Choline. Dietary Reference Intakes for Thiamin,
    Riboflavin, Niacin, Vitamin B6, Folate, Vitamin B12, Pantothenic
    Acid, Biotin, and Choline. 5 Riboflavin: National Academies Press,
    1998, https://www.ncbi.nlm.nih.gov/books/NBK114322/.

52 Niacin. National Institutes of Health, 2022, https://ods.od.nih.gov
    /factsheets/Niacin-HealthProfessional/.

53 Zeisel SH et al: Choline, an essential nutrient for humans. *FASEB J*
    1991, 5:2093–2098.

54 Zeisel SH & da Costa KA: Choline: an essential nutrient for public
    health. *Nutr Rev* 2009, 67:615–623.

55 Norris J: Choline in Vegetarian Diets. 2015, http://extension.oregon
    state.edu/coos/sites/default/files/FFE/documents/choline-rd.pdf.

56 Pantothenic Acid (Vitamin B5)—Uses, Side Effects, and More. WebMD,
    2020, https://www.webmd.com/vitamins/ai/ingredientmono-853/pantothenic
    -acid-vitamin-b5.

57 Vitamin B6. National Institutes of Health, 2023, https://ods.od.nih
    .gov/factsheets/VitaminB6-HealthProfessional/.

58 Biotin (oral routine). Mayo Clinic, 2024, https://www.mayoclinic.org
    /drugs-supplements/biotin-oral-route/description/drg-20062359.

59 Fang H et al: Microbial production of vitamin B12: a review and future
    perspectives. *Microb Cell Fact* 2017, www.ncbi.nlm.nih.gov/pmc/articles/
    PMC5282855.

60 Watanabe F et al: Pseudovitamin B(12) is the predominant cobamide
    of an algal health food, spirulina tablets. *J Agric Food Chem* 1999,
    47:4736–4741.

61 Wells ML et al: Algae as nutritional and functional food sources: revisit-
    ing our understanding. *J Appl Phycol* 2017, 29:949–982.

62 Chen JH & Jiang SJ: Determination of cobalamin in nutritive supple-
    ments and chlorella foods by capillary electrophoresis-inductively cou-
    pled plasma mass spectrometry. *J Agric Food Chem* 2008, 56:1210–1215.

63 Rotter D: Vitamin B12 Daily Requirement. *Vitamin B12 & Health*.
    www.vitaminb12.de/tagesbedarf.

64 Holick MF: Vitamin D: A millenium perspective. *J Cell Biochem* 2003,
    88:296–307.

65　Nehls M: Alzheimer ist heilbar—Rechtzeitig zurück in ein gesundes Leben. Heyne 2015.

66　https://www.norsan-omega.com/algae-oil/;https://sinoplasan.de/en /omega-3-algenoel-dha-epa-100ml; https://www.myfairtrade.com/en/vegan -omega-3-epa-dha.html.

PART VI: THE FUTURE OF A FRONTAL LOBE-WEAKENED HUMANITY

1　Dowbiggin IR: High anxieties: the social construction of anxiety disorders. Can J Psychiatry 2009, 54:429–436; Stein DJ et al: The cross-national epidemiology of social anxiety disorder: Data from the World Mental Health Survey Initiative. *BMC Med* 2017, www.ncbi.nlm.nih .gov/pmc/articles/PMC5535284.

2　Friedrich M & Weik M: Die Digitalisierung macht das Grundeinkommen unumgänglich. *Focus* 23.3.2017, www.focus.de/finanzen/experten/weik _und_.friedrich/arbeitsplaetze-bedroht-die-digitalisierung-macht-das -grundein-kommen-unumgaenglich_id_6761830.html.

3　Reena & Bhatia PK: Application of Genetic Algorithm in Software Engineering: A Review. *Journal of Engineering and Science* (IRJES) 2017, 6:63–69.

4　Cellan-Jones R: Stephen Hawking warns artificial intelligence could end mankind. BBC 2014, www.bbc.com/news/technology-30290540.

5　Angerer C: Neuronale Netze: Revolution für die Wissenschaft? *Spektrum der Wissenschaft* 2018, 1:12–21.

6　Wen H et al: Neural Encoding and Decoding with Deep Learning for Dynamic Natural Vision, *Cereb Cortex* 2017, 1–25.

7　Angerer C: Neuronale Netze: Revolution für die Wissenschaft? *Spektrum der Wissenschaft* 2018, 1:12–21.

8　Dönges J: Computer erzeugt Gemälde aus Fotos. Spektrum.de 16.4.2016, www.spektrum.de/news/computer-erzeugt-gemaelde-aus-fotos/1407867.

9　Listen here: AIVA—"Letz make it happen", Op. 23, www.youtube.com /watch?v=H6Z2n7BhMPY.

10　Nielsen M: Künstliche Intelligenz: Alpha Go—Computer lernen Intuition. *Spektrum der Wissenschaft* 2018, 1:22–27.

11　Eppinger U: Mit künstlicher Intelligenz gegen Depressionen und Angstzustände: Was kann "Dr. Bot" leisten? *Medscape* 4.4.2018, https: //deutsch.medscape.com/artikelansicht/4906868

12 Kermany DS et al: Identifying Medical Diagnoses and Treatable Diseases by Image-Based Deep Learning. *Cell* 2018, 172:1122–1131.

13 Langemak S: Versorgung am laufenden Band: Mit AI verbringen Sie noch weniger Zeit mit dem Patienten. *Medscape* 27.11.2015, https://deutsch. medscape.com/artikelansicht/4904331.

14 Krauth, Olivia: The 10 tech companies that have invested the most money in AI. TechRepublic, 2018, https://www.techrepublic.com/article/the-10-tech-companies-that-have-invested-the-most-money-in-ai/.

15 Chess Network: Google's self-learning AI AlphaZero masters chess in 4 hours. YouTube 2017. www.youtube.com/watch?v=0g9SlVdv1PY.

16 Kurzweil R: *The Singularity Is Near: When Human Transcend Biology*. Viking, 2005.

17 Wolf C: *Vorbild Gehirn*. Gehirn & Geist 2018, 4:56–61.

18 Martin S: AI WARNING: Google chief predicts DIFFICULT TIMES with rise of artificial intelligence. *Sunday Express* 8.11.2017, www .express.co.uk/news/science/877124; Kurzweil R: *How to Create a Mind: The Secret of Human Thought Revealed*. Viking, 2012.

19 Artificial intelligence experts sign open letter to protect mankind from machines. 2015, www.cnet.com/news/artificial-intelligence-experts-sign-open- letter-to-protect-mankind-from-machines; Autonomous Weapons: an Open Letter from AI & Robotics Researchers, 2015, https://futureoflife.org/open- letter-autonomous-weapons/.

20 Woll S: Transhumanism and Posthumanism—An Overview. Or: The Fine Line Between Utopia and Dystopia. *J New Frontiers in Spatial Concepts* 2013, 5:43–48.

21 Martin S: AI robot version of Albert Einstein warns humanity is destroying itself. *Sunday Express* 7.11.2017, www.express.co.uk/news/science/876663.

22 Noordermeer SD et al: A Systematic Review and Meta-analysis of Neuroimaging in Oppositional Defiant Disorder (ODD) and Conduct Disorder (CD) Taking Attention-Deficit Hyperactivity Disorder (ADHD) Into Account. *Neuropsychol Rev* 2016, 26:44–72.

23 Riess H: The Science of Empathy. *J Patient Exp* 2017, 4:74–77.

24 Konrath SH et al: Changes in Dispositional Empathy in American College Students Over Time: A Meta-Analysis. *Personality and Social Psychology Review* 2011, 15:180–198.

25 Decety J: The neurodevelopment of empathy in humans. *Dev Neurosci* 2010, 32:257–267.

26 Watson PJ et al: Narcissism and empathy: validity evidence for the Narcissistic Personality Inventory. *J Pers Assess* 1984, 48:301–305.

27 Niose D: Beware America's Shocking Loss of Empathy. *Psychology Today* 6.3.2016, www.psychologytoday.com/blog/our-humanity-naturally/201603 /beware-americas-shocking-loss-empathy.

28 Streit über Essener Tafel—Dobrindt widerspricht Merkel. *Spiegel* online 27.2.2018, www.spiegel.de/panorama/gesellschaft/essener-tafel-alexander -dobrindt-widerspricht-angela-merkel-a-1195633.html.

29 Popp M: Flüchtlingsdrama im Mittelmeer Abgestumpft. *Spiegel* Online 31.5.2016, www.spiegel.de/politik/ausland/fluechtlinge-europa-ist-abge -stumpft-kommentar-a-1095136.html.

30 Ceballos G et al: Biological annihilation via the ongoing sixth mass extinction signaled by vertebrate population losses and declines. *Proc Natl Acad Sci* USA 2017, 114:6089–6096.

31 Jordan B: Scientists Say Humans' 'Lack of Empathy' is Leading to Global Species Annihilation. *Alternet* 21.12.2017, www.alternet.org /environment/scientists-say-humans-lack-empathy-leading-global -species-annihilation.

32 Riess H: The Science of Empathy. *J Patient Exp* 2017, 4:74–77.

33 Riess H: The Science of Empathy. *Sage Journals*. May 9, 2017. https: //journals.sagepub.com/doi/10.1177/2374373517699267.

34 Baudson TG. The IQ is no longer sufficient. *Spektrum* 15.9.2017, www .spek- trum.de/kolumne/der-iq-reicht-nicht-mehr-aus/1502371.

35 www.medizinfuchs.de/preisvergleich/norsan-omega-3-vegan-100 -ml-san-omega-gmbh-pzn-13476394.html.

36 Google: Market capitalization of Alphabet (Google) (GOOG). October 2024. https://companiesmarketcap.com/alphabet-google/marketcap/

INDEX